# Social Work Approaches to Conflict Resolution
## Making Fighting Obsolete

# Social Work Approaches to Conflict Resolution
## *Making Fighting Obsolete*

Benyamin Chetkow-Yanoov, DSW

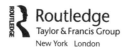

Routledge
Taylor & Francis Group
New York   London

First published by

The Haworth Press, Inc., 10 Alice Street, Binghamton, NY 13904-1580

This edition published 2012 by Routledge

Routledge
Taylor & Francis Group
711 Third Avenue
New York, NY 10017

Routledge
Taylor & Francis Group
2 Park Square, Milton Park
Abingdon, Oxon OX14 4RN

Cover designed by Donna M. Brooks.

**Library of Congress Cataloging-in-Publication Data**

Chetkow-Yanoov, B.
    Social work approaches to conflict resolution : making fighting obsolete / Benyamin Chet-kow-Yanoov.
        p.  cm.
    Includes bibliographical references and index.
    ISBN 0-7890-6035-3 (hardcover : alk. paper) 0-7890-0185-3
    1. Social service. 2. Conflict management. I. Title.
HV41.C442  1996
361.3′2–dc20

                                                                    96-13118
                                                                        CIP

This book is dedicated to the writer of:

## No Complaints*

Love is all I've ever really had.
When love works
it means the world to me, the world
made vivid and young.
                    Once I thought
Love would deliver power, wealth
and endless adoration. Instead
I got more love. Every year. And
the world gets brighter, younger.

---

*I feel that the writer of this poem, whose identity is unknown to me, is a soul-sister or soul-brother. In its original form, "No Complaints" celebrated poetry. I hope that my anonymous colleague approves my substituting the word "love" for "poem" and "poetry" in this dedication.

# ABOUT THE AUTHOR

**Benyamin Chetkow-Yanoov, DSW,** is Professor of Social Work at Bar-Ilan University in Israel. While he has consulted and taught primarily in Canada, the United States, and Israel, he has also conducted workshops in Australia, England, Namibia, South Africa, Thailand, and Sweden. He pioneered a master's level course in conflict resolution at Bar-Ilan University's School of Social Work, and has organized training programs for Israelis wanting to learn conflict resolution skills. He is the author of *The Pursuit of Peace* and has assumed leadership roles in several national government organizations for promoting peace and diplomacy. These include *Partnership*, a voluntary association for creating cooperation between Israeli Arabs and Jews, and *B'Sod Siach*, an organization to facilitate communication between political rightists and leftists. Dr. Chetkow-Yanoov serves as a consultant for Israel's Ministry of Education and is working on its current curriculum project, *Preparing for an Era of Peace*. His professional interests include the dynamics of program implementation, community theatre, systems analysis, voluntarism, leadership among aging professionals, and community social workers vis-à-vis municipal politicians.

# CONTENTS

# Acknowledgments

This book is a product of the stimulation and support of:

- my Jewish and Arab/Palestinian friends–especially those who welcomed me into the voluntary association "Partnership" and those who assisted me in the development of the Neighbors Curriculum as well as in computerizing parts of it;
- my students and colleagues at Bar-Ilan University, who helped me pioneer the first course in conflict resolution at the University's School of Social Work;
- the faculty and staff of the Institute of Conflict Analysis and Research (ICAR) at George Mason University, who stimulated me with their course materials, gave me a place to sit and write, and made my early 1992 visit with them thoroughly stimulating;
- my colleagues, especially Stella Cornelius, at the Conflict Resolution Network of Sydney, Australia, from whom I learned practice truths; and
- my soul-mate Bracha, who continues to edit all my English-language writings and to make critical suggestions for improving them.

# Introduction

## *EXPERIENCING PEACE TREATIES IN MY LIFETIME*

I consider myself very blessed indeed. In my 25 years in Israel, I have personally experienced the signing of two peace treaties–the Camp David Accord between Israel and Egypt, and the treaty between Israel and the Palestinian Liberation Organization. In fact, on September 13, 1993, my wife and I postponed a social work committee meeting in order to watch the TV coverage of the signing of the Declaration of Principles (which led to the Oslo I treaty in 1994).

I came away with a new and deepened appreciation of the long and secret process that made the final signing possible. I felt proud that Israel's political leaders had outgrown their military backgrounds in order to take risks for peace. True, many people on both the Israeli and the Palestinian sides found the prospect of peacemaking frightening, but many more of us began to hope that the hostilities of the past 100 years might finally be de-escalating. We celebrated that compromises were possible–enough for both sides to feel that the outcome was worthwhile.

It became obvious that the peace process was also helped along by some voluntary efforts well outside formal governmental auspices. Apparently a multitrack effort is essential to break the habits and policies of so many years. I was also impressed with the sophistication of the coverage of the event in many newsmedia–enough to wonder how we might enlist the media as partners in future conflict resolution efforts.

All these topics, as well as some others, are elaborated in this book. I hope my readers will get as excited about conflict resolution as I have become. If there is to be peace on earth in the coming century, it must begin with each one of us personally.

## *MY START IN THIS FIELD*

My interest in conflict resolution has evolved over many years. The seed was planted in Vancouver, Canada, when I was beaten up for being the only Jew in my seventh grade class (those racist jeers still echo in my memory). Toward the end of the 1960s, my family settled in a racially changing neighborhood of Indianapolis, Indiana, where my wife and I became involved in founding an interracial neighborhood association. Though I had not caused the problem of racism, I wanted to have a part in not handing that problem on to my children's generation.

Living in an interracial neighborhood introduced me to victim behavior. I noticed that some of my new black colleagues/neighbors acted like an "Uncle Tom" with me, and a few of them were so full of rage that it interfered with their own self-interests. Nevertheless, we found ways to learn about each other, and gradually some of us came to trust each other enough to work together on such matters of common interest as preventing violations of zoning or promoting enrichment programs at our unsegregated local school. Although some social distance remained between us, we did find the human-ness that was our common heritage, occasionally even celebrating holidays together.

The personal benefit from this experience was twofold: my igno-rance about other people who had suffered prejudice and victimiza-tion (as had the Jews) was lessened. I learned not to fear human beings who were different from me. When we understood things differently, or when we disagreed about some neighborhood activ-ity, we worked hard to find mutually acceptable resolutions. I felt good when my friends trusted me enough to take me to meetings in the black ghetto of Indianapolis.

In the summer of 1971, my family moved to Israel. As new immigrants, we were involved in getting absorbed in the culture (including the experience of the Yom Kippur War) for the next six years. The existence of an Arab-Jewish conflict did not penetrate our consciousness (on a personal level) until we were electrified by President Sadat's visit in 1977. His risk taking, and the subsequent mediation of Dr. Henry Kissinger, made a deep impression on me. I remember being amazed that some of my Israeli-born friends were deeply afraid of the prospect of peace in the region and unwilling to trust any Arabs–even those who were fellow citizens of Israel. As a professional social worker, I was motivated to look for explanations, and while I searched, I developed a growing sense of urgency.

In 1979 my wife and I joined (and eventually became leaders in) a voluntary peace organization called Partnership–dedicated to creating conditions of coexistence between Israel's Jewish and Arab citizens. Our Indianapolis experience proved helpful–we knew how to remedy our ignorance, and being involved with strangers did not trigger fear reactions in either of us. In fact, we were upset when some of our Jewish colleagues and neighbors interpreted our working for Arab-Jewish coexistence as a Jewish disloyalty. We were confused by the fact that they, as part of a people who had survived a holocaust, could talk about Arabs in stereotypic and racist terms.

During more than a year of workshops, we learned some Middle East history, did self-awareness exercises, practiced new skills in running mixed groups, visited Arab homes and were hosts in return, and learned how to manage our feelings in confrontational situations. In all this, my resolve was strengthened by my growing friendship with a veteran military man turned peace educator–Wellesley Aron. Through his pioneering efforts for peace within Israeli and international Rotary, as well as his demonstrating that peace topics could be taught within a Tel Aviv public school, he inspired me deeply (Silman-Cheong 1992).

Gradually, I found myself calling on my social work background and theoretic concepts from the social sciences to try to explain what happened in my Arab-Jewish coexistence work. Similarly, examples of coexistence behaviors began to appear in my teaching. I quickly became aware of the many parallels between my experiences as a Jew and the African-American or Palestinian experience as persecuted minority peoples.

As an adult social worker, and after many painful rejections as a young Jew, I became convinced that conflicts were being generated by intergroup clashes of values, feelings of fear, outbursts of accumulated rage, resentment of long-continuing stigmatization/victimization, continuing imbalances of power/resources, and dangerous patterns of unmet human needs. I felt that conflict resolution had to address emotional factors urgently if any difference could be made in Northern Ireland, South Africa, Israel, Cambodia, India, Rwanda, or the former Yugoslavia.

At local and international professional conferences, I found that many of my Israeli experiences could be generalized (especially when they were conceived in systems-analysis terms). My experiences proved useful at workshops and institutes that I was invited to give in Canada, England, Holland, Namibia, South Africa, Sweden, Switzerland, and the United States.

During the 1980s, I became an active member of the World Council of Curriculum and Instruction (WCCI). As an outcome of writing and editing two peace curricula for Israeli schools, and of participating in a number of WCCI international conferences, I discovered the growing literature of conflict resolution, and that the subject had become a legitimate academic discipline in a number of European and North American universities. I began to make contacts with colleagues in this field. In 1992, I spent part of a sabbatical at the Institute for Conflict Analysis and Resolution (ICAR) of George Mason University (Fairfax, VA, USA), and with The Conflict Resolution Network of Sydney, Australia.

As my new friends welcomed me into their backyard, I sensed that an input of social work insights might enrich the conflict resolution field. This book constitutes my effort in that direction.

## SUMMARY OF THE BOOK'S CONTENTS

The title of this book clearly implies that, although some conflicts may serve useful purposes, all "fights" are negative–and should be eliminated. Throughout this book, fighting always connotes conflict escalation, a desire to destroy the other side rather than be reconciled in the future, and the use of violence in order to win.

Part I of this book focuses on "conflict" as a problem of interest to the helping professions. Causes of conflict are the focus of Part II. The focus of Part III is on ways to cope with conflict and teaching conflict resolution skills. Section IV includes summaries and recommendations. Specifically:

Chapter 1 opens with a look at similarities and differences between *solving problems and resolving conflicts.* A seven-phase model of problem solving is presented. Implications for the practice of social interventions in conflict resolution follow.

Chapter 2 begins with a look at my experience in Arab-Jewish reconciliation in Israel, and at some of the contributions of my social work background to understanding conflict and violence. The chapter introduces a *systems model of conflict analysis*–focusing on four interacting components of any conflict. Specific combinations of these components give rise to five types of conflict outcomes.

In order to understand one of the causes of conflict (Part II), Chapter 3 explores the contribution of *value clashes* to generating conflicts.

Chapter 4 examines the dynamics of *segregation, integration, and coexistence* relationships as outcomes of complex power conflicts between establishments and various disadvantaged (minority) groups. Of the above three models, coexistence is suggested as useful for de-escalating intergroup conflicts.

Chapter 5 looks at the behavior of *victims and victimizers.* In general, victimized people and groups are seen as major contributors to the perpetuation and escalation of conflicts.

Having presented some ways to analyze conflict, Chapter 6 (at the start of Part III) focuses on a range of social work *intervention strategies* that derive from the analytic models presented in the previous chapters. Ten steps are suggested for helping victims to free themselves from repeating conflict-generating behaviors.

Chapter 7 examines a number of *professional roles* necessary in order to accomplish the kinds of interventions described in the previous chapter.

Chapter 8 reviews trends in the evolution of voluntary conflict resolution efforts and gives brief consideration to possible roles for *citizen volunteers as conflict resolvers* in personal, organizational, and intergroup settings. This chapter analyzes, within an ambivalent Israeli society, the vanguard function of one Arab-Jewish voluntary organization. Other examples of voluntary efforts are also included.

Chapter 9 opens Part IV by elaborating a number of ways in which education and social work specifically could contribute to the conflict resolution field. Assuming that relevant *knowledge, attitudes, and skills can be taught* in every country, the chapter goes on to describe a diversity of available programs for teaching conflict resolution to nursery, elementary, high school, university, and adult audiences.

Chapter 10 looks at a number of *factors that enhance or impede the resolving of conflicts* in a variety of tension-laden settings. The summary includes the posing of a new model for conflict resolution. The chapter closes with a set of recommendations.

# PART I:
# CONFLICT AS A SOCIAL PROBLEM

Chapter 1

# A Systems Model
# for Solving Problems

## INTRODUCTION

Social work has been described as a profession that engages in solving social problems and in resolving conflicts (Parsons 1988). We might do well to remember that problem solving and resolving conflicts can produce both positive and negative outcomes. Some social workers, like physicians, intervene in order to lessen inadequate (or "sick") behaviors and to help the sufferers become cured of them. Other social workers see problems and conflicts as opportunities for growth, or as leverage for bringing about desirable change.

We will try to define both topics in this opening chapter. First, let us look at social problems and what is usually meant by the term "problem solving." We will do the same for "conflict" later in this chapter.

## LOOKING AT PROBLEMS

In order to bring the above two perspectives together, we might define problem solving as an activity in which a person or group:

1. focuses on a human or social condition that is considered incomplete or normatively unacceptable;
2. is dissatisfied with or disturbed by this incompleteness; and
3. feels ready to make an extra effort in order to try to remedy the situation–that is, to bring or return it to a condition of completeness or acceptability.

For example, perfectly normal people who want to improve their chess-playing skills often sit at home and practice solving chess problems. Similarly, welfare ministry bureaucrats, dissatisfied that a large percentage of our population lives in poverty, have designed programs of neighborhood renewal. Those problematic situations that do get attention are seen as challenges rather than pathologies. They trigger emotional or value-laden responses that motivate us to do something about them, and we become willing to participate personally in solving a problem or resolving a conflict (Rosenheim 1976).

Problems may arise from at least two types of causes. The first type, like hunger or jealousy, is based on a lack of something essential (e.g., food or love). In social work, such problems are labeled "needs." Solving such problems may seem relatively easy. They can often be eliminated by supplying what is missing. Just as adoption is a solution for orphaned children, income is the answer for unemployed breadwinners and schools are an antidote for illiteracy. In many Western countries during this century, social services were created to take care of unmet needs of citizens caught up in rapidly urbanizing and industrializing societies. Since social services try to supply what a person or system lacks, these personnel operate from a position of relative strength.

A very different type of problem is caused by the accumulation of unwanted surpluses. Thus, problems such as overweight, lung congestion, or violence are caused by eating too many sweets, breathing industrial wastes, or the proliferation of gang wars. Such problems are usually seen as negative —so much so that the causal factors must be stopped or modified if the problem is to be solved. This may require the problem solvers to fight against very powerful vested interests that profit from preserving the status quo. Here, the intervenor is likely to become engaged in confrontation.

Both problems arising from scarcity (e.g., lack of income and skills in impoverished neighborhoods) and those caused by unwanted surpluses (e.g., growing violence in an inner-city slum) can be seen as either pathologies to be treated or as challenges to be solved (and perhaps prevented). In either eventuality, solving social problems is very complicated (Rittel and Webber 1973). Problems are often hard to define, and their causality may be unclear (i.e., multiple). People stop working on problems when they run out of time or money, rather than because they have solved them.

The presenting problem may itself be the outcome of another unsolved problem. Often, discrepancies can be explained in a number of ways, and zero-sum solutions (where somebody wins at the expense of others) come back to haunt us. Solutions for social problems are seldom right or wrong, but rather are judged by how well they lessen suffering or satisfy needs under specific interactional or environmental conditions. Sometimes the adequacy of a solution is judged by how well it conforms to the goals or values of the ruling (local) political party.

## A PROBLEM-SOLVING MODEL

Figure 1.1 shows how problem solving in the helping professions can involve us in a seven-phase model.

### A. Initial Problem Situation

At the start, the model articulates the nature of the initial problem situation (which may or may not include conflict). We could, for example, focus on a teenager who is already getting into trouble as a result of her growing addiction to drugs, or on a group of parents from a middle-class neighborhood who fear for their children's safety when the children cross a high-traffic road on their way to school. We usually supplement our initial understanding of the problem situation with a subprocess of objective information-gathering and direct observation.

### B. Clarifying the Causes of the Problem

Before taking action, professional persons enrich their efforts with theory-derived knowledge or models of why people or groups behave as they do. With a daring guess (or hypothesis), we are now required to assess whether the drug addict is, for example, suffering from blocked opportunities or from neglectful parents. Similarly, we could verify that street crossing is dangerous for inexperienced

FIGURE 1.1. A Problem-Solving Model

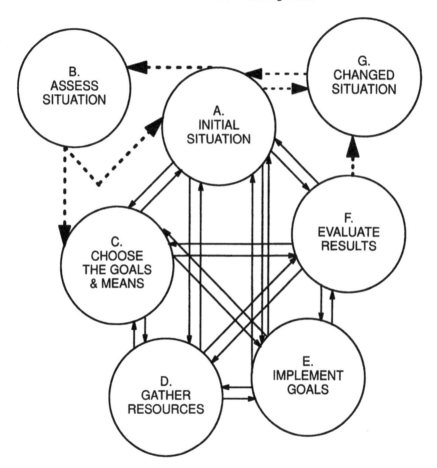

nursery and first-grade children. With such a combination of facts and theory, we identify factors that cause the problem or make its solution urgent.*

---

*Of course, effective professional intervention should address its efforts toward preventing or diminishing the causes of the problem—not simply toward minimizing the symptoms or dealing efficiently with later outcomes.

## C. Choosing Goals and Means

Once a hypothesis regarding causality is formulated, we must establish action goals. Although we want the goals to be logical outcomes of the problem to be solved, goal determination is often constrained by the expressed desires of those suffering from the problem, by our own professional values, by the resources available, and by our awareness of community or societal priorities. In every case, we expect goals and means to remain intertwined and compatible.

So, after as much preparation as possible, we must decide what we intend to do about the problem and what interventions are likely to bring about the desired change. We can decide:

1. to do nothing;
2. to try to rehabilitate the sufferers and/or their families–perhaps through casework counseling;
3. to do crisis intervention by operating a telephone hot-line;
4. to try to prevent specific problems from developing altogether (e.g., run an afterschool club program rather than have kids play on the streets, where they are all too often enticed into using drugs); or
5. to strengthen healthy behavior of normal children (e.g., by sending them to summer camp).

We are likely to favor goals that can be implemented inexpensively and with minimal opposition.

Since goal setting includes recommending the most effective method we know for intervening, we might decide to help an addicted teenager receive rehabilitative treatment (correction personnel might also want her to be punished). For the parent group, we might include raising funds to make possible the implementation of a safety education program at the school and the installation of a traffic light (or a pedestrian overpass), so that the children can cross the road safely. If implementing these interventions do not pose special budgetary problems, they are likely to be approved (see phase "E").

Goal and method determination, important as they are, are not enough. The process must include making the goals operational, so that project outcomes can be evaluated. Appropriate change-targets are to be specified, and criteria are determined for judging (in the future) whether the goals have or have not been attained. For example, we may decide that local delinquency is due to lack of supervised free-time settings for children of working parents. If, as the method of intervening, a local elementary school opens a youth club for its pupils during the after-school and early-evening hours, criteria of its success might include:

1. Children from many classrooms and from the surrounding neighborhood become members, and renew their memberships after one year;
2. The total number of members increases over a specific time period;
3. The children find club activities attractive, show signs of having fun, and even suggest additional activities for their group;
4. Statistics indicate a lessened incidence of delinquent behaviors (e.g., less noise, fights, property damage, drug use) in the neighborhood;
5. The club proves so popular that, upon request, its doors are opened to population groups like retirees, during the morning hours when the children are in school;
6. The club opens a well-attended junior-leaders training program, and its graduates start social clubs for younger children who would otherwise play on the streets (and most likely get into trouble); and
7. Extension versions of the club program start up in apartment-house basements or unused public shelters, and visitors from other parts of the community duplicate the model in their school districts.

After a predetermined period of time, objective evaluators will be able to determine whether the above conditions were or were not brought into existence (see phase "F" in Figure 1.1).

### D. Gathering and Preparing Resources

Once goals have been determined philosophically and operationally, phase "D" (see Figure 1.1) can begin. Both the client and action systems, being as creative and efficient as possible, gather together the resources necessary for implementing the strategies and technologies identified in phase "C." They might apply for a grant from a charitable fund, ask for contingency funds from their municipality or a governmental ministry, or decide to pool resources with a number of social services. Since few projects depend on one set of resources alone, project staff may also be required to function as coordinators of the resource providers. The staff will also be responsible for reporting to the donors how each particular donation was to be used.

### E. Taking Action to Implement the Plan

Once the resources have been located, the staff begin to act — hopefully in accordance with the systems' goals. Professional and administrative persons use resources to produce desired changes in themselves or in others within a relatively short period of time. During this implementation phase, records should be kept of all intervention efforts and outcomes, until (and even after) the change goals are reached. A formal monitoring (in writing, statistics, or videos) of decisions made and of actions undertaken is part of sound implementation.

### F. Evaluating Results

After the intervention methods have been operational for a designated period of time, a process of outcome evaluation (phase "F") should take place. Data about the current situation must be studied and compared to the goal statements made in phase "C." If the young lady remains clean of drugs after completing her rehabilitation program, we might infer that her problem has been solved. If there is a significant drop in delinquency generally and in drug use specifically, our after-school program is worth continuing.

Similarly, if no children have been involved in car accidents on their way to and from school after a full year, it would seem that the problem has been solved. Evaluation might also reveal whether the children had learned about safety in a cognitive way, or whether they had internalized new skills that enable them to recognize and avoid traffic dangers.

Evaluation could focus both on whether a problem has been solved successfully and on whether the solution was efficient or expensive.

## G. Follow-up

Evaluation implies follow-up. Thus, we will want to check if what has been done produced a significant change from what had been the initial problem-environment (in phase "A"). If we find a lower incidence of girls using drugs and if the school's traffic accidents decrease and these decreases remain stable for a period of two years, we may judge that the goals have been achieved and the problem has been alleviated or solved.

What has been learned might prove useful for solving similar problems in other communities –thus becoming a contribution to the development of knowledge and ensuring that those who come later do not have to "reinvent the wheel." The knowledge might then be incorporated into a new policy statement regarding the project's continued operation.

## LOOKING AT CONFLICT

As mentioned above, the problems that the helping professions encounter are often exacerbated by conflict. Conflict usually refers to disputes and disrupted relations between individuals or groups who have incompatible or rival:

1. purposes (e.g., freedom and independence vs. domination and exploitation);
2. value-based norms (e.g., whether abortion is desirable or shameful);
3. needs (e.g., for land, security, recognition, or respect);
4. feelings (e.g., fear and hatred vs. trust and love);
5. opinions (e.g., our region should be "cleansed" of inferior races); or
6. interests or desires (e.g., two nations wanting to control the same waterway).

The Conflict Resolution Network of Australia suggests that we should be alert to the possibility of conflict when interpersonal or intergroup relations are accompanied by increasing discomfort, hostile incidents, and misunderstandings. If relationships involve tension and repeated crises, not only are we dealing with a conflict, we may also be facing its escalation toward violence (Cornelius and Faire 1989).

Prolonged fights are characteristic of the destructive relationships between Catholics and Protestants in Northern Ireland, the Serbs and Croats in former Yugoslavia, blacks against blacks in Africa, and the recent genocides in Europe and in Cambodia. What happened between whites and Afro-Americans in the United States, and what is in process between Israelis and Palestinians during the time of this book's publication suggests that nonviolent ways of conflict resolving do exist. As is elaborated elsewhere in this book, when we can break the habits of centuries (which sanctioned fighting and warfare in times of conflict), we will discover that there are forms of conflict that serve useful purposes.

In the meantime, we can identify a number of specific conditions that give rise to conflicts or cause them to escalate into various forms of violence. For example, an uneven distribution of power often leads to conflicts that escalate. The same is likely when rivals feel required to compete for what they define as indivisible or scarce resources. Sometimes, conflict results when the success of one party precludes other parties from achieving a similar success (win/lose outcomes). This may, in fact, trigger a cycle of violent revenge-efforts by the losers.

In other words, conflicts may be analyzed according to their symptoms (e.g., discomfort, crisis), their causes (e.g., unmet needs, power asymmetry, victimization), or their outcomes (e.g., the five types of conflict discussed in Chapter 2).

## *SOLVING PROBLEMS*
## *AND RESOLVING CONFLICTS*

Problem solving and conflict resolving are complicated by the nature of the people viewing or defining them. For example, it is important to realize that different people, with different values or pragmatic interests, are discussing the same situation. We may, for example, be given very different versions of a conflict in an impoverished neighborhood by its long-time residents, by nurses of the local public health clinic, or by members of the city council (Germain 1991; Kluckhohn 1951).

A similar situation occurs when the observers tend to view a problem objectively or subjectively. When the condition or its solution can be expressed in clearcut or quantitative units, the problem is viewed objectively. Researchers are especially happy when they can count precisely how many people in a community suffer from cholera, are homeless, seek help against depression, or are killed in automobile accidents every week. Similar accuracy is possible regarding levels of income or of education, or regarding the number of pension-receiving engineers over age 85.

On the other hand, how do we describe objectively the suffering experienced because of ignorance or war? Have we objective ways to record the helplessness caused by racism, fraud, or rape? We do not yet know how to measure the suffering of families whose loved ones were killed in the daily slaughter on the roads. Some scholars have a very limited view, contending that if a problem cannot be defined in measurable terms, it does not exist (Hudson 1978).

It is indeed difficult to demonstrate that a problem exists (or has been managed effectively) when its presence/absence, frequency, magnitude, or duration are accompanied by strong feelings of indignation among those who study the problem. In such conditions, those responsible for intervention might well identify with what Charles Lindbolm (1959), a professor of economics at Yale University, wrote that we often must be satisfied with merely muddling through.

Similarly, tensions or crises that mirror conflicts of interest might be classified as objective, but conflicts based on unmet needs (e.g., jobs by members of a racial minority) become utterly subjective and are often not negotiable. Problems that do not involve representatives of all relevant factions are basically unresolvable. However, most conflicts, because they involve interaction with other people or organizations, cannot be resolved alone. They may well require third-party assistance with problem solving in order to move toward reconciliation, or to reverse the process of escalation.

Often, technical solutions to a problem are insufficient, and we must also repair the wounded relationships that are responsible for long-lasting opposition or hatred (Parsons 1991; Ury 1993). It follows that problem-solving and conflict resolution, though not identical, do have much in common.

## IMPLICATIONS

The above discussion implies that problem solving, although often very complex, *can* take place. Based on the contents of the following chapters, we will also show how many conflicts can be resolved. Both the problem-solving and the conflict-resolving processes rely on gathering facts and matching them with theoretic knowledge in order to define the problem or conflict and in order to diagnose causality. Unsolved problems tend to lead to outbursts or escalation of conflict. Advocates of both the above-mentioned processes favor participatory rather than coercive interventions, see helpful outcomes resulting from trust relationships, and stress the utilitarian or win/win basis of long-lasting solutions.

It is often claimed that we do not solve conflicts. If we are patient, and can nibble at them persistently (i.e., re-solve them again and again), we might keep them under control. Truly successful interventions against conflict cause the situation to undergo a transformation, so that the conflict-causing problem ceases to exist. This topic is pursued in a later chapter of this book.

Chapter 2

# A Systems Model
# for Analyzing Conflicts

## INTRODUCTION

The promotion of peace education has become increasingly popular in diverse scholarly disciplines since the early 1960s. As a community social worker and a social-work educator, I have been trying
since 1963 to relate my professional knowledge of nonviolent social
change processes to the issues of war and peace. In fact, I was
stimulated by Eileen Younghusband's 1963 focus on the rapid and
almost universal social change that resulted from technological
innovations connected with the industrial revolution. Although
these innovations greatly increased humankind's muscle and thinking capacity, she found "no such means to enlarge his . . . heart, and
. . . this widening imbalance in man's development means that the
benefits conferred by his mind may be negated by the infantile and
uncivilized responses of his emotions."

Like many others, I began with the assumption that service disciplines such as social work and the behavioral sciences are capable of
reducing this gap between ultra-sophisticated technology and
social-emotional immaturity (Addams 1922; Crane 1986; Hamilton
1958; Konopka 1953; Lundy 1987). My sense of urgency was deepened by a growing awareness of the destructive relationships that
have developed between diverse ethnic peoples all over the world.
For example, *Newsweek* of September 16, 1991 reported that Corsi-
cans wanted to leave France, Yugoslavia's ethnic groups were on the
verge of a civil war, Russia was becoming a "dis-Union," and
French and Flemish speakers were in conflict again in Belgium.
Similar tensions were erupting in Spain, India, South Africa, the
Sudan, Ireland, Canada, Nigeria, and Israel.

Humankind will, indeed, be in serious trouble if we let our generation's mistakes, injustices, and inappropriate attitudes become the inheritance of the next generation. Our successors must be prepared for a world vastly different from the one in which we grew up. For example, they must function in a world where electronic media has eliminated the isolation of illiteracy and distance. Today, the use of violence as a tool of political policy has become dysfunctional. We must prepare the next generation for effective coping with uncertainty, as well as give it the confidence to abandon old solutions that no longer work. Countries will have to learn how to operate as pluralistic or multiethnic societies. If groups or peoples are to survive into the twenty-first century, the ways of coercion (oppression, racism) and of pressure-cooker integration would have to be replaced by those of coexistence (Amir and Sharan 1984; Chetkow-Yanoov 1990; Grier and Cobbs 1968).

The Jewish tradition contains a wise saying: "Who is the greatest of heroes? He who converts his enemy into his friend" (Avot D'Rabi Nathan 23). This idea should be used to communicate to our youth a nonmilitary sense of bravery. High-risk occupations require physical skill and courage, but the supreme heroes are persons who, like Mahatma Gandhi or Martin Luther King, risk their lives in order to communicate with those who disagree with them, and do this by using the power of empathy or love.

My desire to start teaching conflict resolution was strengthened by President Sadat's visit to Jerusalem in 1977. During the subsequent peace treaty negotiations with Egypt, a cautious optimism began to be felt among some Israeli Jews. Others resisted a shift to a nonhostile relationship with Arabs after years of enmity. They also resisted a thaw in their relationships with Arab fellow citizens of Israel. I wanted to deal with the fact that many of my Jewish Israeli colleagues found the prospect of peace frightening.

## THE CONTRIBUTION OF SOCIAL WORK
## TO CONFLICT RESOLUTION

Since social work has long engaged in conflict resolution, it has much to offer to students of this field. Practitioners know, for example, how fear, anger, or guilt affect human behavior as well as physical or mental health. They know that a healthy person, group, or nation may indeed need to be assertive in order to initiate a new action or be creative. An exaggeration of the same energy can, of course, produce hostility, victimization, or violence—especially if basic needs are left unmet or are violated.

Fighting seems likely to erupt, between individuals or nations, when they cease communicating with each other. Social workers know that material wealth, beyond a flexible standard of decency, does not make for well-being. Unlike Moliere's miser, people who give of themselves and of their possessions feel stronger than those who hoard luxuries, comforts, money, or military technologies.

Being powerful enough to dominate others does not guarantee peace. A loser's acquiescence does not create a trust relationship—only dependency and resentment. In the Middle East, as in other parts of this planet, people who have suffered oppression for many years tend to internalize a victim self-image. During their lifetimes, victims tend to be at the core of many continuing conflicts. In fact, we have become increasingly aware of the very small separation between being victimized and becoming a victimizer of others (see Chapter 5). When we understand this pattern of linked behaviors, we can seek ways to exchange the self-image of victim for a more healthy one (Chetkow-Yanoov 1985; Danielli 1985; Dimsdale 1980; Shipler 1986; Silverman 1975).

## WHAT DO PEOPLE FIGHT OVER?

In simple terms, most conflicts emerge around a limited variety of situations or issues. The following types of conflict usually lead to fighting, and if appropriate intervention does not take place, may escalate into violence.

People and groups seem to fight when they want to:

1. achieve or retain exclusive control over something scarce, valuable, or prestigious—such as gold, oil, uranium, rivers, mountain passes, sovereignty over land, ocean ports, cash crops, trade routes;
2. dictate the agenda for other persons or groups (sometimes called coercion)—such as, to win elections, to exert pressure on

the authorities (e.g., by lobbying), to get special consideration (as would the supervisor of a large staff group), or to exploit a minority group;

3. defend themselves or their group against threats to honor, importance, or survival. In other words, healthy human beings will make extraordinary efforts to satisfy such unmet needs as those for food and shelter, security, identity, recognition, or actualization. This seems especially relevant to the outbursts of ethnic tribalism in the early 1990s;

4. preserve or justify the rightness of their values, beliefs, or ideology—as seen in the exaggerated behavior of most fundamentalists or fanatics;

5. lessen the tension between some of their different roles—e.g., one person coping with the competing demands of being a mother to young children, wife of a partner, assistant manager in a bank, and chairperson of a voluntary organization (Goodbread 1993);

6. get revenge or special compensation for real or imagined past insults, exploitation, or suffering—as is typical of the behavior of most long-time victims or victimized groups; and

7. attract attention to oneself or to an issue that seems neglected—as is typical of the way the political opposition courts the mass media in any working democracy.

## POSITIVE AND NEGATIVE ASPECTS OF CONFLICT

Actually, some forms of conflict seem essential for normal living. Perhaps the first experience of this is just before birth, when the unborn child has to push hard to get out of the contracting birth canal. Without a modicum of friction, we could not stand, walk, or run (Coser 1965; Deutsch 1973; Warren 1972).

Let us review some of the *positive aspects* of conflict:

1. Actual competition between manufacturers seems essential if factory laborers are not to be exploited, consumers do not have to pay higher prices, or taxpayers do not suffer. In a one-party government, or when (in a multiparty system) there is no opposition, democratic elections lose their significance.

2. Conflict can raise public awareness about what is going on in the world, especially if the events are covered by the news media.
3. Confrontation and conflict can lead to an increased effort to solve problems or to achieve advances in technology.
4. Conflict stimulates self-testing and reality testing.
5. The philosopher Hegel claimed that any normal point of view (or thesis) generates its own antithesis, and that the two eventually integrate into a new synthesis. Thus, a measure of conflict is essential to the process of creativity.
6. Conflict requires contact between the parties, often making it more desirable than apathy or isolation.
7. Limited conflict is one way to achieve short-term lowering of tension, experience immediate relief, or work out aggressions.
8. Like a catalyst, conflict produces results quickly–as when marital discord hastens a couple's movement toward divorce or reconciliation.
9. Conflict may lead to a redistribution of economic, political, or social resources.

In the same manner, let us look at some of the *negative outcomes* of continuing or escalating conflicts:

1. Although conflict can focus attention on certain issues, it may do so at the expense of distracting attention from other important issues or events, thus leading to costly neglect. This is especially wasteful when conflict is used to divert attention from specific targets or to conceal a scandal from public attention.
2. It is a mistake to think that participation in a conflict leads to group cohesion. Struggling against a common enemy or danger may cause temporary group adhesion, but as soon as the pressure eases, people usually return to their former interests and rivalries.
3. In an attempt to preserve our mental health during periods of conflict, we often dehumanize (or demonize) our opponents– e.g., by claiming they are "primitive," they stink, or there is no one to talk to on the other side. This helps free us from responsibility for the scapegoating, exploitation, or violence that we perpetrate against our opponents.

4. It is dangerous to forget the suffering or humiliation of (weak or wounded) opponents who lose. They are likely to demand compensation or revenge at some future time.
5. Conflict of interests may raise the costs of a planned project, especially if it leads to duplication of efforts or continuing rivalry (e.g., competition between management and unions preventing a cooperative effort to save a faltering business during a time of economic recession).
6. Healthy assertiveness that is unfairly restrained may well erupt into violence at a later date and then prove expensive to all parties in the conflict.

The focus of this book is less on preventing or restraining conflict than on what methods may be used to prevent or reverse the negative outcomes listed above.

## *CONFLICT AS HIGH-ENERGY INTERACTION*

Some scholars conceptualize conflict as the negative extreme of a consensus-dissensus range of human behaviors. At the one end are such behaviors as *consensus,* agreement, goodwill, sharing, joint problem solving, cooperation, and compromise. In the middle we find behaviors such as *competition,* disagreement, bargaining, negotiation, persuasion, rivalry, protest, confrontation, even clashes (all within the approved norms of the culture/society within which they take place). At the disapproved extreme are violence, destruction, norm-violation, coercion/repression, humiliation, murder, and war (Brager and Specht 1969; Kramer 1969; Warren 1965). The three types are summarized in Figure 2.1.

For the purposes of this book, conflict is seen as a form of human interaction, usually between at least two persons or groups who are committed to traditions, goals, interests, or ideological positions that:

*Are incompatible.* If the satisfying of the demands/desires of one participant clearly excludes that possibility from all other participants (e.g., groups who believe in abortion vs. those who advocate the embryo's right to be born), serious conflicts are probable.

*Prevent all participants from satisfying their basic needs.* Serious conflicts are probable when people (e.g., Kurds in Turkey) feel they must act very aggressively in order to survive (Burton 1991).

*Are accompanied by powerful emotions.* In situations rife with fear, jealousy, rage, hatred, or desire for revenge, some form of healing has to take place so that the parties (e.g., the Serbs and the Croats of former Yugoslavia) do not push each other into increasingly violent conflict.

I agree with those scholars who contend that *conflict is the result of healthy assertiveness.* Like Freud's id, assertiveness is seen as a basic energy that enables human beings to survive in a hostile environment, to discover truths by means of risk taking, to be creative, to show initiative in unpredictable situations, and even to trust others enough in order to work with them cooperatively. Some assertive behaviors are indeed fear induced or connected to protecting

FIGURE 2.1. Three Aspects of Conflict

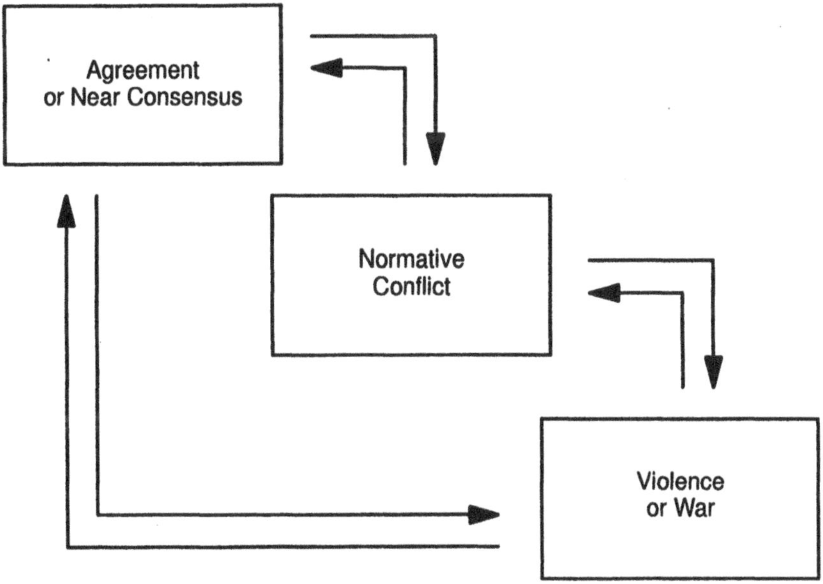

territorial ownership. Others seem essential for relating to the other sex, having and raising children, etc.–that is, are instrumental. In the twentieth century, men such as Mahatma Ghandi and Martin Luther King taught us how to use assertive power nonviolently for achieving planned social change (Moyer 1971; Smoker, Davies, and Munske 1990).

I also suggest that specific interpersonal and environmental *conditions can turn assertiveness into destructive aggression*. For example, interethnic or tribal rivalry (not necessarily a "bad" thing) that has continued unchecked for hundreds of years is likely to produce the agonies now typical of Yugoslavia or Rwanda. Over time, the rivals are likely to become psychologically or ideologically closed, and to see their world in dichotomous terms: us (the just) vs. them (the evil ones). Such attitudes encourage a conflict to escalate into violence. Similarly, lack of attention to the needs of large groups of human beings, gross imbalances of power/resources among rival parties, or the rise of dictators such as Stalin or Idi Amin, cause the intensity of conflicts to rise significantly.

These topics are discussed throughout the rest of this chapter, and are illustrated in Figure 2.2.

Under such conditions, a basic human energy is distorted into something negative and used to dominate or control others–often by such means as scapegoating, victimization, or violence. Such negative uses of our interactive energy often lead to outcomes such as child abuse, wife beating, slavery, or genocide. Other parts of this book argue that sophisticated interventions can de-escalate most conflicts away from destructive aggressiveness back toward healthy assertiveness.

## *A SYSTEMIC PARADIGM OF CONFLICT*

The recognition of conflict, and the practice of conflict resolution, are important goals for all the helping professions. New definitions of human nature, and analyses of conditions of affluence rather than scarcity, have produced a shift in conflict theory away from simplistic single-cause pictures toward the use of systemic paradigms (Burton and Sandole 1986). A systems approach to analyzing conflict,

FIGURE 2.2. Conflict as Outcomes of Assertiveness or Aggressiveness

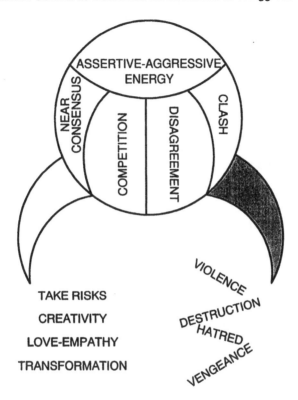

and to conflict resolution, can indicate how certain types of conflicts may be functional or dysfunctional for a human system.

People who rely on systems-based analysis are able to grasp total or holistic situations rather then deal with detached fragments. System thinking allows us to become sensitive to:

1. the drawing of a clear, arbitrary boundary that defines the social system (e.g., a nuclear family);
2. sets of persistent, interdependent (horizontal) relationships among the components of the system (e.g., sibling relationships within the nuclear family);

3. the beliefs, sentiments, symbols, and control mechanisms that reinforce a system's coherence and persistence (e.g., love, belonging to a specific religion);
4. the context or environment outside of a system's boundaries (e.g., nursery school services in the neighborhood);
5. vertical interrelationships between components of the system and components of other systems in its environment (e.g., family adults who serve on the local school's Parent-Teachers Association); and
6. continuous interchange of relationships/resources among components, the system, and its environment.

A systemic outlook also helps us see how many components interact—both impacting on all other components and being influenced by them simultaneously (Chetkow-Yanoov 1992).

If we rely on a systems model of conflict, the intervention ideas in this book can be applied equally well in clinical, family, group, community, organizational, or international settings. This model suggests that a systemic approach is helpful for analyzing all types of conflict and for choosing professional interventions appropriate to dealing with one component by itself or with combinations of them.

## FOUR COMPONENTS
## OF ALL CONFLICT SYSTEMS

When analyzed within a comprehensive components-system-environment model, all conflicts seem to include at least four basic components (see Figure 2.3).

As in all open systems, each component is simultaneously making an impact on the other three and being influenced by them. This being so, the interaction between basic components remains relevant to any type or size of conflict. Although other components may also be operating, these four are present to a lesser or greater extent in every conflict.

### Duration of Tension or Pressure

We must become informed of the duration of a conflict, and know how it impacts on the level of tension/pressure that has built up

FIGURE 2.3. Four Causes/Components of All Conflicts

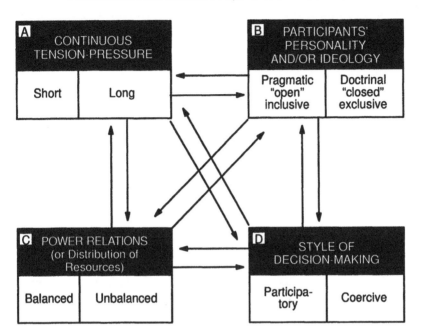

among its participants. Short conflicts are relatively easy to settle; long-lasting ones are, however, much more difficult to handle. Under conditions of strong pressure or tension from a system's environment, most individuals or groups experience a crisis. Normally, people in crisis feel helpless or inadequate for, say, a few months–and then begin to recover, as they do after mourning the loss of a loved one. Short crisis periods often prove beneficial to a person's growth and may help a person to innovate new solutions to existing problems. The situation becomes very complicated when the crisis persists for a long period of time and causes significant erosion of mental health. Exhausted persons cope poorly, resulting in more stress.

Human beings, in situations of unceasing tension, often defend their actions by simplifying the world into dichotomous "we" vs. "them" divisions. They tend to abandon the middle ground in various continua. As their thinking becomes more and more polarized, their functioning tends to become more closed and they rely on a coercive style of decision making and tend to project blame onto other participants. Without significant relief from the tension, they may indeed experience burnout, leave the community/environment, or escalate a conflict into violence.

---

*Hypothesis:* The shorter the duration of a conflict, the less likely it is to escalate into violence.

---

### Personality or Ideology of the Participants

It seems to me that long-lasting conflicts are often accompanied by a change from pragmatic, inclusive, playful, decentralized, open behavior to a humorless devotion to purity of principles, centralization, exclusiveness, and secrecy (Avruch and Black 1991; Hoffer 1951; Sanzenbach 1989). Later analysis will suggest that certain combinations of emotions (such as fear and anger) tend to push human systems toward closedness and even fanaticism. Participation in long-lasting conflicts makes the boundaries of the systems involved less and less permeable.

In recent history, such closed behavior was exemplified by the action style of the late Ayatollah Khomeini. Similarly, when the very conservative Barry Goldwater was a candidate for the presidency of the United States, he came up with the slogan "Better dead than Red." In such closed persons or systems, participants tend to become more and more fanatic and to see the world in dichotomous categories. Alternatives disappear, and even bystanders must decide if they are "for me or against me." Generally, the situation worsens if the participants are also ignorant of the characteristics and the norms of the opposing group. Then both sides fall victim to rumors, generalizations, and stereotypes, and tend to function in a decidedly self-righteous style. Lack of communication between opponents can be both a contributing cause and a result of conflict.

Closed-minded participants, or tightly closed systems, are likely to dominate decision making and exclude others as unworthy of consideration. When closed-minded persons also have a great amount of power, they can frustrate most efforts to resolve any conflict in which they are participating, or rationalize the use of violence against a persistent opponent.

---

*Hypothesis:* The more "open" one or all the participants are, the less likely that a conflict will escalate in the direction of violence.

---

### Distribution of Power or Resources

Basing themselves in political science and worldly realities, scholars such as Lingas (1988) or Weingarten and Leas (1987) emphasize the centrality of power in situations of long-lasting conflict. The course of a conflict is influenced by competition for power, authority influence, or control.

In fact, there are two basic kinds of power:

1. coercive or manipulative types of power–physical, military, political, economic, governmental, legal, organized masses of people, bureaucratic-administrative, and skills in public relations or marketing; or
2. social types of power–such as personal commitment, gender-based charm, the normative prestige of elders, the capacity to project empathy or caring, and the ability to motivate people to take part in sharing or cooperation (Etzioni 1975).

These distinctions are central to later analysis of an establishment's relations with minority groups (see Chapter 4), and of conflict resolution interventions that seek to create power balances (see Chapter 6).

Purnell (1988) and Eisler (1987) stress the differences between power arrangements that are symmetric (all rivals are of similar strength, power is shared) or not (one side is very strong, the other is weak). Actually, most of the social problems that concern the helping professions may be analyzed as the product of power imbalances or the coercive uses of power. Poor people, stigmatized minority groups, children, widows, orphans, disengaged old persons, or those who live in ghetto slums suffer because they lack sufficient "clout" to require the local establishment to deal with their unmet needs (Parsons 1991). Corrective efforts often include strengthening the weak (e.g., leadership training, listening to grievances with empathy, financial assistance, activating the news media on behalf of the impoverished neighborhood), or creating a system of legal checks on the overly strong.

In the days of the great empires, the strong ruled and the weak were conquered and/or exploited. Today, too, a powerful elite can control things paternalistically or manipulate the social control mechanisms of its subordinates. If, however, a strong party is too oppressive, members of the dominated side may become embittered, increase the impermeability of its boundaries, or resort to violent rebellion.

---

*Hypothesis:* The more symmetric the power or resources between participants in a conflict, the less a conflict is likely to escalate into violence.

---

### Style of Decision Making

From organization theory, we learn about three styles of decision making: denying the necessity for making any decision at all, deciding coercively what everyone must do, or inviting all relevant parties to participate in making a decision. Denial (usually done in a relatively closed system) is not recommended, primarily because it eliminates any possibility for improving the situation. The other two styles are elaborated and contrasted in Table 2.1.

Domination achieves quick results at someone else's expense (i.e., it creates win/lose outcomes). However, such victories tend to be unstable, as well as more and more costly to sustain. They also generate resentment that contributes to conflict intensification. Domination is usually rooted in suspicion, fear, contempt, and secrecy–conditions for attaining obedience. Further, oligarchic priv-

TABLE 2.1

| COOPERATIVE STYLE | COERCIVE STYLE |
|---|---|
| The basis of pluralistic democracy. | Typical of totalitarianism, domination, or oligarchy. |
| Seek common denominators, tolerance, coexistence, and participation. | Retain exclusivity and segregation, clear restrictions on minorities. |
| Faith, good will, and empathy are basic; expect and promote cooperation, sharing, consensus, coordination, exchange, negotiation, compromise, horizontal relations among diverse interest or pressure groups, partnerships. | Suspicion, enmity, and contempt are basic; expect and promote cutthroat competition, making every effort to win, selfishness, capitulation of subordinates (vertical relations), obedience to orders, little actual opposition. |
| Useful for creating a basic level of trust relations and interaction. | Useful for restoring order rapidly after the onset of a serious crisis. |
| Requires a two-way or open flow of communications. | Relies on a one-way flow of communication or secrecy. |
| Based on equality, or one standard for everyone. | Based on the continuation of privilege, superiority. |
| Encourages self-help and citizen participation. | Relies on master-plans made by bureaucrats and experts. |
| Conflict is managed through joint problem-solving. | Conflict is managed by means of arbitration. |

ilege often causes bureaucratic manipulation, rivalry for control, or racist exploitation of the weak.

On the other hand, participatory coalition making constitutes the basis for cooperation, and makes for win/win outcomes. Widening opportunities for rivals to participate jointly in a system's production activities or to enjoy part of its outputs (e.g., food-buying cooperatives, interdisciplinary committees, or multiparty coalitions) constitute a sound basis for conflict resolution. Although participation processes take longer than coercion, the benefits of client involvement in agency decisions, or in self-help processes, have been amply documented. The participatory style is usually accompanied by ideological openness, power sharing or exchange, and a readiness to coexist with others in a complex pluralistic world (Chetkow-Yanoov 1991b).

---

*Hypothesis:* The less decision making is coercive, the less likely that a conflict will escalate in the direction of violence.

---

We recommend to conflict resolution personnel that, to the extent that they have control over such matters, they try to limit conflicts to as short a duration as possible, help all disputants to be or to remain as open-minded as possible, strive for a balance of power or resources among the disputants, and engage the parties in participatory decision making as much as possible. Other combinations tend to make conflicts escalate in the direction of increased tension and/or violence.

The model appears to be relevant to conflict situations of all sizes–whether between individual adults in a violence-plagued family, between rival neighborhood gangs, between the former establishment and the people of Rumania, between religious factions in India or Ireland, between right wing and left wing political parties, between pro-life and pro-choice movements in the U.S. abortion controversy, between Jews and Palestinians in Israel, between the African-Americans and whites in New York City, or between rival black tribes in South Africa.

## OUTCOMES:
## FIVE TYPES OR PHASES OF CONFLICT

Lingas (1988) defined social work as a harmony-building profession, noting that client crises are often caused by unresolved conflicts and blocked communications. Other conceptualizations of conflict include those of Chin and Benne (1969) who analyze the process of change as the product of efforts to achieve tension reduction, Weingarten and Leas' (1987) proposal of a five-stage mediation model for marriage counselors, and Warren and Hyman (1966) who discuss consensus and dissensus in cases of community change. Actually, to examine conflict fully, we should examine a range of behaviors, from consensus (i.e., no conflict) to various forms of violent fighting (Avruch and Black 1990; Burton 1991,

Clark 1990; Parry 1987). Although many theory-derived models are in use to explain the idea of conflict, the five-level one presented here is recommended.

Analysis of combinations of the above four conflict components enables us to discover five basic types of conflict outcomes. For example, we might work simultaneously with two components: (a) symmetric or asymmetric power arrangements, and (b) flexible/ closed ideologies or personalities of participants. The other two components, shortness of duration and a cooperative decision-making style, correlate strongly with flexibility. Similarly, long-duration conflicts and coercive decision making match up with closed-mindedness of the participants.

Thus, five types of conflict outcomes can be derived by means of a four-cell table, using power symmetry/asymmetry and flexible/ closed-mindedness (see Table 2.2).

When these two variables are analyzed together, we are able to clarify the characteristics of five kinds of conflicts or five phases of any particular conflict. These appear to be:

## *Near Consensus*

A situation of flexibility/inclusiveness and balanced power arrangements usually gives birth to consensus, that is, to cooperation and sharing between power equals. Each participant or group is likely to be happy with the outcome, having attained something desirable that it could not have achieved alone. For example, consensus is the ideal basis for a family decision (after full discussion) regarding what to do together during summer vacation. Even in this atmosphere of general agreement, a participant can ask for clarification, request additional discussion time, argue logically, or insist on an open vote. If this process of cooperation produces results that seem worthwhile to all the parties involved, cooperation will continue, and serious conflicts are unlikely.

Basic agreement or consensus is likely under conditions of trust, equality of resources, open communication, and high levels of participation (see elaboration in Chapter 7). After the tension and excitement generated by a full discussion of an issue, those assembled are able to act in harmony to solve their problems (as is done at Quaker meetings). Such a situation results in a win/win

TABLE 2.2. Five Types of Conflict Outcomes

| Actual Power Arrange-ments | Personality or Ideology of Participants | |
|---|---|---|
| | Flexible and Inclusive | Closed and Rejective |
| No Unit Has a Monopoly (.5 / .5) | 1) NEAR-CONSENSUS (win/win)<br><br>Between equals.<br><br>High participation.<br><br>e.g., NATO, voluntary associa-tions, Oslo Agreement, Neighborhood committee. | 3) DISAGREEMENT (compromise)<br><br>Reluctant collaboration between same-strength groups.<br><br>e.g., coordination, city plan-ning, coalitions, councils, European Union. |
| One Unit Has a Monopoly (1 / 0) | 2) COMPETITION (win/lose)<br><br>The strongest competitor wins today.<br><br>The weaker side submits tem-porarily.<br><br>e.g., olympics, elections, foot-ball league, advertising, drama festival. | 4) CLASH (lose/win)<br><br>Normative control by the pow-erful.<br><br>The weak submit.<br><br>e.g., bureaucratic administra-tion, a lawsuit, police enforcement, "persuasion" by monopolies. |

5) DESTRUCTION/VIOLENCE (lose/lose)

The players use violent means.

The weak are victimized.

e.g., neighborhood gangs, army conquest, Stalin's government, civil war, racist genocide.

outcome, since all parties end up with what they wanted. This group is often characterized as nearly conflictless, or in a state of whole-ness basic to a definition of peace.

### *Contest or Competition*

Flexibility together with power imbalance create competition. In this situation, the "rules of the game" require that the stronger side win. If the weaker side cannot invoke arbitration, initiate a lawsuit, or boycott the proceedings, it will have to find long-term ways to strengthen its position or settle for less than it really wants. As in competitive sports, the stronger player wins today, but in tomorrow's game, today's loser may rally and take back the prize.

In competitive situations, one participant is expected to lose and to accept the loss. This type of conflict can be gentle and normative, or it can, as in some big business rivalries, be quite vicious. In delicate situations, the stronger party (e.g., the Interior Ministry) may act in a restrained way so as not to risk harming its ongoing relations with local (e.g., municipal) decision makers. However, it often uses considerable pressure (such as offers of budget allocations or threats of arbitration) to convince the locals to follow in the Ministry's footsteps.

### Difference or Disagreement

Closed-mindedness within a power balance gestates disagreement or differences of opinion. When highly principled players are not strong enough to dominate, they negotiate or compromise. Most cooperation, as in political party coalitions, takes place because each of the parties involved lack sufficient power to operate independently (that is, their participation in joint activities is ambivalent). In most parts of the world, persons responsible for urban planning are also experts at compromising reluctantly.

Cooperation within difference is likely when the parties connected to some issue disagree on some things, but their differences remain partial. They find it worthwhile to act together regarding those aspects of the issue on which they do agree, and have sufficient items in common to cooperate with each other or to come to a mutually satisfying compromise—in which all parties get less than they originally wanted, but nobody suffers a total loss. Case conferences, where the workers of a number of social agencies negotiate ways of working together to rehabilitate one multiproblem family, are often rooted in this sort of environment.

### Dissensus or Clash

Closed-mindedness and power monopoly produce dissensus, as exemplified by the open clashes around the Anglican decision to ordain female clergy, fights over ideological purity, or nonviolent protest rallies. In such situations, the strong party attempts to dictate the outcome, or undertakes to implement its program unilaterally. The others might oppose openly or engage in deliberate confrontation. However, all parties continue to respect accepted norms or rules of the game, and the side that loses acquiesces for the time being (Specht, 1969).

In this type of conflict, coercive power is used not only in order to win, but also to dominate the situation permanently. Partisan members (of one faction) may use confrontation or disruptive tactics, initiate a lawsuit, create a powerful lobby, or join the opposition in order to get their way. This level of conflict is very strong, and permanent losers may feel victimized. However, all parties adhere to the norms of mutual respect and the possibility of reconciliation. Deliberate nonviolent violation of societal norms may take place in order to focus attention on what one side sees as gross injustice. Conflicts between rival political parties (especially before elections) or between labor and management groups, are typical of this situation.

### Violence or War

When one or both parties in a conflict decide that resolution has become impossible and are ready to go beyond the accepted norms toward harming or destroying their opponent, they have escalated to the level of violence–exemplified by the gang wars in the neighborhoods of *West Side Story.* When the weaker side is opposed in principle to compromise (as are fighters for freedom rebelling against colonial regimes), the price of keeping order escalates. In the event that the weaker side feels compelled to seek revenge by using violence, the stronger party engages in backlash, and the cost to each side increases. Ultimately, both sides may end up losing status, money, power, or lives (Chetkow-Yanoov 1976 and 1987; Warren 1972).

Violence may appear in an institutional format (e.g., sexism, racism, impoverishment) or directly (e.g., abused children, terrorism, torture, war). This form of conflict is not only costly to all sides, but it may, as in Somalia, actually destroy the environment and the society in which it takes place.

The impact of the combination of power arrangements and closed-mindedness on conflict dynamics is further illustrated in Figure 2.4.

FIGURE 2.4. The Phases of Conflict Escalation

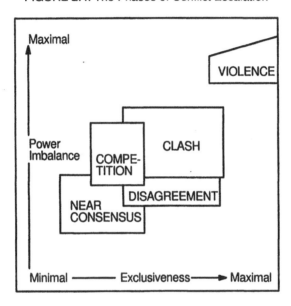

If the above (consensus to violence) model is used to illustrate five phases of one conflict, it is well to remember that neither escalation nor de-escalation proceed in a simple linear way. Complex combinations of closedness and unbalanced power seem to increase the risk of violence. In an era of rising expectations and snooping television, deprived populations may resort to violence if they see no hope for improvement in their immediate future.

The challenge is to devise intervention strategies appropriate for de-escalation from violence. We may, therefore, want to learn how to open up a closed system, or how to create power balance, in order to increase the chances of resolving specific types of conflicts.

## *SUMMARY*

In this chapter, a systems model was introduced, focusing on four interacting components of all conflicts. Specific combinations of two components, system flexibility or closedness and symmetry/ asymmetry of power arrangements, gave rise to five types of conflicts. Interventions geared toward dealing with the various components, as well as with the five types of conflict, are elaborated on in Chapter 6.

# PART II:
# SOME SOCIAL CAUSES OF CONFLICT

Chapter 3

# Conflicts Generated by Unmet Needs and Clashes of Values

## SOME CONFLICTS ARE GENERATED BY UNMET NEEDS

Philosophers, theologians, psychologists, anthropologists, social workers, and political scientists have all written extensively on the idea of human needs (Clark 1990; Towle 1965). In principle, they claim that a diversity of elements or conditions are so essential for human survival or for wholesome growth and maturation that normal people, in a state of healthy tension, make extra efforts to get these needs satisfied. In order to satisfy such needs, behaviors are stimulated that lead to satisfying the needs in ways sanctioned by local values and norms.*

If basic human needs are not satisfied, personal pathologies or social problems tend to develop (e.g., those of post-Vietnam war veterans in the United States). The post-traumatic behavior of long-victimized individuals or population groups constitutes one clear example of the cost of unmet needs.

Abraham Maslow (1954) created a hierarchic model of needs, as follows:

1. The most basic are *physical needs*–for food, water, shelter, clothing, and the like. In the novels of Charles Dickens, we saw how normally honest but poor men risked stealing bread from bakeries when they or their children were starving.

---

*The connection between needs and values has long been recognized by anthropologists (see Lee 1959). It is discussed in a later section of this chapter.

Human beings generally have a strong drive for self-preservation, so that meeting physical needs becomes part of survival. Of course, meeting these needs requires that food is grown in the environment and that local stores have staple foods to sell, housing be available for rental or purchase, drinking water is not poisoned with sewage, etc. Once these basic needs are satisfied, normal persons are able to devote their efforts to satisfying nonmaterial types of needs.

2. According to Maslow, most people then strive to satisfy their *security needs*–that is, a normal need for physical safety (from harm, danger, or accidents) as well as for economic security (by means of a job, a steady income, or reliable social and commercial insurances in their environment). People whose security needs are met learn to trust others. Most people desire security both in an immediate sense and for their future years. When this need remains unsatisfied, situations of uncertainty generate high levels of anxiety and fear. Such people tend to subscribe to obsessively conservative values.

3. Normal human beings next try to satisfy their *social or identity needs.* We all need to feel that we belong somewhere, and are accepted members of a family, small group, an organization, or an ethnic population. Feelings of love, affection, and closeness are involved, and these contribute to a person's growing sense of identity. Persons born into stigmatized minority groups may have serious difficulties getting this need satisfied in a normative way. They may even be ashamed of the ethnic group into which they were born, and want to leave it. Thus, when the in-group with which others identify them does not satisfy their social need adequately, they may have to satisfy this need by associating themselves with reference groups that they admire but cannot actually join. Frustrated identity needs are sometimes satisfied by forming irrationally strong attachments to specific geographic territories (as Jews and Palestinians have done in the Middle East), or by seeking membership in a religious cult.

4. Maslow claims that normal human beings also have a need for *respect, status, recognition, or esteem.* On the basis of the value placed on achievement, we become confident, indepen-

dent, and motivated to take risks in order to learn. Of course, self-respect is as important as achieving a positive reputation (or prestige) through feedback from others. Reciprocal role relationships, like those between student and teacher or parent and child, are basic to satisfying this need. When healthy channels for satisfying this need are blocked, many people try to acquire respect or esteem by means of buying expensive possessions or living in an exclusive neighborhood.

5. Highest in Maslow's hierarchy is the need to make progress toward one's full potential, i.e., for *fulfilling or actualizing one's total self.* In order to satisfy this sophisticated need, we must live in an environment containing enough opportunities to enable us both to find an occupation we are fitted for and to enjoy the satisfactions of doing it well. Actualized people are open to new experiences, do not fear the unknown, enjoy improvising creatively, and are able to go beyond existing categories to integrate or synthesize ideas from diverse sources (Maslow 1968).

Maslow himself suggested that the order of needs is not absolute, and people may work on more than one need at a time. Although we can all think of one or two exceptional people who overcame deprivations, all the need levels must be satisfied in order to become a fulfilled person. Needs that remain basically unsatisfied may stall growth or create a receptivity for antisocial values and behaviors.

Students of conflict resolution claim that many continuing conflicts are caused by the unmet needs of the participants (Burton 1991; Parsons 1991). Thus, satisfying the parties' needs for dignity and security in a war-torn region may have to precede negotiations over territory or the distribution of resources (Rothman 1989). When, as in the parts of former Yugoslavia, opponents do not recognize each other's unsatisfied needs for identity, belonging, or participation conflicts tend to continue or to escalate.

Matters may be exacerbated as much by improperly satisfied needs as by needs that are not satisfied at all. In an unpublished conference paper, Pietila (1982) points out how much of today's consumption tries to satisfy nonmaterial hungers with material goods—to no avail. If, for example, Jewish security in the Middle

East is based on having a big army or a wide buffer zone, defense expenses may skyrocket but they will not create a sense of security. The factors that create security, according to Maslow, are other than powerful armies or large occupied territories. Similarly, when the need for esteem is based on buying expensive possessions or cars, there will never be enough money, and the person involved may actually turn into a miser. In other situations, ethnic groups who hunger for prestige may satisfy that need by victimizing some other group. Their self-respect is not based on anything qualitative, but rather is derived from arbitrarily declaring themselves to be "better" than a group they are scapegoating.

When the gap between needs and level of need satisfaction is small, deprived individuals and groups can usually survive (see Figure 3.1). However, when the gap gets large enough to seem intolerable, deprivation leads first to unrest, then to a values shift, and finally to the eruption of a conflict that escalates into violence (Davies 1969).

FIGURE 3.1. Conflict as a Product of Declining Need-Satisfaction

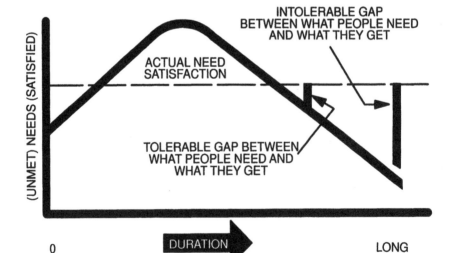

## *INTRODUCTION TO VALUES*

Values are the conceptual-moral-behavioral standards that human beings believe to be proper or right for themselves and for other members of their society. Expressed as customs, ritual behaviors, institutional arrangements, definitions of basic needs, or moral commandments, values indicate what a society defines as especially significant. Values determine the answer to such a question as: Was the truth revealed in the past, is it found in the here and now, or is it to be discovered in the future? Similarly, values give us a paradigm of human nature as evil, neutral, or good from birth. Within any specific society, basic values preset our behavioral expectations as well as our ways of thinking. They determine our paradigms of the universe, of the good society, as well as of human behavior (Kluckhohn 1951). Values help us determine, for example, whether sex is lovely or dirty, whether working is good and idleness is not, whether stealing is bad, whether respecting old persons is good or unimportant, whether women should be subordinate to men, what is beautiful or ugly, and what behaviors are liberal or conservative.

As the family, religion, the schools, and other social institutions contribute to our socialization, values become transmuted into behavioral norms as well as beliefs. They become the basis of what every society calls "normal" human behavior (Levy 1973). Adult human beings who are members of a professional association accept a value-derived code of ethical behavior. For example, social workers believe that healthy human beings can change and develop, that all human beings need love and empathic attention from others in order to develop, and that personal information divulged during therapy sessions must be kept confidential–and are trained to act accordingly.

Values also direct our definitions of a problem (see Chapter 1). If a criminologist believes certain violent behaviors to be deviant and deserving of punishment, a psychiatrist might see the same behavior as a symptom of a sickness (resulting from lifelong impoverishment) requiring therapeutic help, and a social worker may view those behaviors as a sign of healing (e.g., a previously apathetic client who now expresses anger in very aggressive behavior). Values lie behind our certainty that, for example, the spread of literacy or of democracy are progress rather than mere change.

As the result of years of socialization and of reinforcement by social control mechanisms, values are both charged with strong emotional energies and, within any given society, accepted as self-evidently true (Avruch and Black 1990; Free and Cantril 1967). An attack on values might make people feel uncertain and even afraid–as if they were being attacked personally.

In an agency setting or within the same community, holders of contradictory values (e.g., economists, planners, political leaders, and helping-profession staff persons) often get into conflicts of principle. As we shall explore in the next section of this chapter, these people might disagree about the nature of the problem as well as about what might be the best way to cope with it–based on a lifetime commitment to specific values (Chetkow-Yanoov 1967; Merton 1957).

## *VALUE-BASED ROLE CONFLICTS*

Goodbread (1993) argues that many conflicts arise between incompatible roles as well as between human beings or groups with rival power aspirations. In this vein, a conflictual outcome is likely when:

1. a person is frustrated by being unable to change roles (as are members of stigmatized minority groups);
2. someone occupying a number of roles simultaneously cannot manage the incompatible obligations of these overlapping roles (e.g., of mother, wife, president of a philanthropic club, and vice president of a real estate office); and
3. persons occupying similar or overlapping roles are unable, because of clashing value commitments, to work cooperatively.

It seems that many historical clashes, such as the Thirty Years War between Roman Catholic and Protestant Christians in Europe, originated in rival definitions of "good" and "evil."

A modern equivalent is the often violent conflict between those who support abortion rights (pro-choice for the pregnant woman) and those who advocate an unborn child's right to survive (pro-lifers). The latter, in their efforts to save babies, sometimes even burn down abortion clinics or attack doctors who work in them (Hoffer 1951; Richan 1991). Emotionally intense value-derived behaviors are characteristic of partisans on both sides and underline the serious difficulties in trying to resolve such conflicts.

At the municipal level, community social workers often find themselves in conflict with local political leaders–again because of differing (and often incompatible) value commitments. Social workers contend that goals will best be achieved after a time-consuming process of citizen participation, that project goals and means must be compatible, and that significant plans must take into account the social needs of a weak population. Local politicians hold quite different views. They argue that: goal implementation must be rapid if things are to get done within their term of office; all controversial projects must be open to bargaining and compromise; any means that succeed are legitimate; participation in goal setting should focus on the needs of powerful voters; and social services are funded in order to strengthen the political stability of the local community.

When occupants of these two roles must work for the public good, to create service-related social policies or to manage controversial issues, they may find themselves in serious conflict (Chetkow-Yanoov 1978; Katan 1974). A case in point is what happened in the Canadian province of British Columbia during the years 1972-1975 (Kavic and Nixon 1978; Turnbull 1975). Two social workers headed a socialist political party that won a majority of the seats in the provincial legislature, constituted the government, and enacted an impressive amount of social legislation during their three years in office. However, despite the party's remarkable social accomplishments, it was not reelected. Insufficient attention to the day-by-day requirements of party politics proved its undoing. The party was true to the social work principles of its leaders, but lost power because of the leaders' political naivety.

Community settings may be more complex than the above simple dichotomy would suggest. In most North American cities, three value-oriented groups compete with each other: fund raisers/allocators (political and community leaders), social planners (helping professionals), and social agency directors (professional administrators).

Their value orientations differ as follows:

| FUND RAISERS-ALLOCATORS | SOCIAL PLANNERS | DIRECT-SERVICE ADMINISTRATORS |
|---|---|---|
| Raise enough funds each year. | Create a balance of services. | Expand to serve more clients. |
| Punitive view of dependency. | Prevention of dependency. | Give help to all who are dependent. |
| Current services are adequate. | Document existing unmet needs. | Current services are inadequate. |
| Desire administrative efficiency. | Desire consent and cooperation. | Desire for agency autonomy. |
| Preserve the status quo. | Plan for directed social change. | Work for agency self-maintenance. |

Some of the above value-based goal orientations may be common to more than one of the three role-players, but they generally predict how that decision maker will behave when called upon to implement or block fund allocations. For example, a study of decisions regarding health and welfare services in metropolitan Indianapolis, United States, during the early 1960s indicated that United Fund leaders were likely to be against routine expansion of social services, preferring to keep agency spending at its current level. On the other hand, expansion requests were made persistently by agency directors and their lay supporters. These stands often generated conflicts among the community's decision makers. Both groups were at times very impatient with the long-range and objective focus of the Social Planning Council's staff (Atherton 1990; Chetkow 1967; D'Antonio 1966).

## IMPLICATIONS

In Shakespeare's era, as mirrored in his play *Henry V,* the clash of mighty opposites (such as the French and the English nations) was resolved by one of them winning the Battle of Agincourt. Although this raw-power approach is still popular, it has not produced long-term resolutions for the many conflicts taking place in various parts of planet Earth. Unresolved clashes over basic values continue to escalate into violent fights.

We would do well to search for other ways to settle serious, value-based disagreements. In the abortion clashes described above, a woman might be persuaded to complete her unwanted pregnancy if the expenses of her pregnancy were subsidized (including her legal and psychological/spiritual counseling), if adoption arrangements were completed directly from the hospital, or if a reliable group of peers could offer her support through the entire period. On the other hand, people with strong pro-life values must cease attacking doctors or destroying clinics. With the help of a skilled mediator, perhaps they would meet with the other side, negotiate and brainstorm together, and agree to specific genetic and moral conditions under which an abortion might be acceptable.

Professional and volunteer ways to cope with various types of conflict are found in Chapters 6 through 8.

Chapter 4

# Conflicts Generated
# by Establishment-Minority Relations

## *LIVING IN TODAY'S PLURALIST REALITY*

In a world that seems to be getting smaller every day, public institutions, metropolitan areas, even entire countries seem less and less homogeneous. Many countries have, in fact, become transformed from one-culture societies into ethnically or linguistically pluralistic ones. The operation of the European Common Market, and of the United Nations itself, seems to be suffering because of the rampant heterogeneity of today's world. We no longer go out to the "Far" East–as if Europe were the center of the world; instead, we travel to Thailand or to Japan. Ethnic or cultural minority groups are no longer willing to be exploited economically. Often a national identity (or peoplehood) is no longer synonymous with citizenship in a geographic country (Hoffman 1982; Rothman 1989).

After centuries of elitistic rule, we find serious minority-majority conflicts in such diverse countries as Belgium, Canada, Germany, India, Iran, Ireland, Liberia, South Africa, Spain, the United States, the former USSR, and Yugoslavia. The lot of gypsy, oriental, or black population groups continue to be difficult throughout the entire world. In light of the disruptive and costly consequences, business as usual is becoming risky.

## *ASYMMETRIC POWER RELATIONSHIPS*

Establishment-minority relations are not usually based on population size, but rather on predefined inequality. The majority, regardless of its numerical size, is seen as the right-and-proper group to command most of the available power and resources, to make policy, to control the enactment and enforcement of laws, as well as to determine the rules of the power game itself. Local values and norms sanction a reality in which minority populations continue to have few resources and meager services.

People who are different from the establishment group (based on distinctions of skin color, religion, language, ethnic origin, culture, or historic experiences) are seen as deserving to be ignored or rejected (Chetkow-Yanoov 1990; Frazer 1962). In other words, the "inadequacy" of minority group persons is prejudged; it has little to do with their standards of behavior or their effectiveness in performing specific roles.

In this conceptualization of power asymmetry, the weak group is very restricted as to what it can do to improve its position. Minority group members continue to be seen as:

1. different, strange, nonnormative;
2. morally inferior, primitive, not quite human;
3. undeserving of equal rights;
4. fit only for doing society's dirty jobs; and
5. unclean, evil, corrupting.

Again, these judgments are not based on empirical facts. They are, at least in part, the outcome of a continuing ignorance about the true nature of the minority group.

The elite's coercive behavior is often rooted in an unrecognized fear of the very minority population that it is exploiting. In the days of historic colonial empires, the above ideas served as ideological justification for exploiting weak groups or nations. This was justified in terms of perverted Darwinism, credos such as "the white man's burden," or early capitalism's need for cheap labor and captive consumer populations.

When weak groups were isolated, they tended to conform to the desires of the majority group, and even tried to be like them. Today, because growing literacy and access to television have made oppressed groups aware of what they are missing, they are much less conformist, and today's exploiters may well have something to fear.

## THREE PATTERNS
## OF INTERGROUP RELATIONSHIPS

Over the past few thousand years, three basic patterns of interaction between strong and weak groups have emerged, as follows:

### Segregation

In segregated societies, legal and physical separation (i.e., isolation) of the designated minority group is the rule. Usually this means that the elite group lives well, while subordinate groups are neglected, dehumanized, rejected, and frequently victimized. Because of a clear asymmetry of resources among the parties involved, the powerful establishment often uses segregation to divide, conquer, and exploit (Anda 1984). The minority group usually has significantly fewer public and social services, and the few existing ones are of poor quality. Its members must compete harder for jobs, rights, and common amenities than do majority group persons.

Because the establishment controls public education and the mass media, and most of the public lacks normal social contacts with minority group persons, members of the minority continue to be seen in stereotypes (generalized categories that allow for few exceptions). This enforces ghettoization, overidentification with the aggressor by members of the oppressed group, and self-hatred. On the other hand, when such victimization is seen by the minority as unjustified, it leads to a rising tide of anger, violence, and terrorism, and then to counter-terrorism backlash—as exemplified by black-white relations in South Africa or the civil war in Spain during this century (Grier and Cobbs 1968; Fattah 1981). Today, subscribing to the segregation model becomes more and more expensive for the establishment—as the English learned the hard way in Ireland or the Israelis learned in the West Bank.

An oppressed minority group does not necessarily lapse into shame and apathy. It often compensates for the harshness of reality by giving itself a sense of being an unrecognized actual or spiritual elite (Kosmin 1979). As explained in Chapter 6, if members of an exploited minority population eventually win freedom and come to power without dealing with their accumulated rage in a healthy way, their thirst for vengeance may cause them to scapegoat others even more harshly than they had been scapegoated in their own past (Shamir and Sullivan 1985). The cost to everyone of intertribal wars in many black African countries, after they became independent of colonial masters, has been very high.

In summary, a segregated society invests heavily in policing or social control. It will be stable, organized, and, as in fascist Italy, the trains run on time. Its decision-making will be centralized, authoritarian, and fast. In it, strangers are controlled, exploited, or eliminated.

### Integration

In this alternative to segregation, the majority group makes a deliberate effort to resocialize or acculturate the minority. The latter is expected to shed much of its cultural uniqueness (i.e., to become deculturated) and to assimilate into the majority culture. Actually, the majority group often absorbs some minority culture characteristics into its way of life, becoming a bit more like the minority group it is trying to absorb. As in the United States of the late nineteenth and early twentieth centuries, immigrant populations were seen as minority groups. They were expected to integrate (i.e., to disappear) over a reasonable period of time–under what has been called "pressure cooker" or "melting pot" conditions (Watts and Hughes 1964; Young 1967).

At first, integration results in both groups modifying or discarding some of their former characteristics, gradually becoming more and more like each other. Ultimately, both groups merge into a new homogeneity. In theory, integration is supposed to improve the lot of the minority group. As it becomes more and more like the majority, its members qualify for the same rights as everyone else. Actually, total integration may destroy the informal network of mutual aid previously typical of minority group society, and it causes members of the minority group identity problems and persistent feelings of loss.

Self-respecting members of the minority group usually try to maintain their uniqueness despite the temptations that integration poses. They tend to marry only persons of their own group, send their children to private (ethnic) day schools, and keep certain ceremonies in private (Eaton 1952; Clark 1990). Minority persons develop a special kind of humor that pokes fun at themselves and also at the majority group, in acceptable ways. Some groups, such as today's Armenians or Basques, refuse to integrate altogether.

Since an integrated society aims for the tranquility of homogeneity, it will have to invest heavily in education and resocialization services. Its decision making is based on normative consensus, and may be much slower than in segregated/coercive settings. Strangers (often immigrants) are seen as raw material to be put into the societal pressure cooker so that their uniqueness can be shed as quickly as possible. Such a society may also tend toward minimal risk taking, or conservatism.

## Coexistence

Based on the reality that most countries are ethnically heterogeneous, the proponents of coexistence argue that it is acceptable (for you) to be different (from me) as long as we both respect each other's uniqueness and rights within a flexible range of normative citizen behaviors. Of course, coexistence involves more than living next to each other and not interfering in each other's lives. Ethnic pluralism or diversity is valued because it can lead to mutual appreciation and enrichment. Basically, all persons have equal rights, and there is no penalty for multiple loyalties. According to the values of coexistence proponents, some ethnically based nonconformist behavior (i.e., uncertainty) is wholesome for a pluralist society.

In order for coexistence to succeed, all groups admit their interdependence and accept responsibility for one another's basic survival. Intergroup relations based on self-respect as well as respect for others usually turn into mutual enrichment. Very different groups may do some activity together on a basis of pragmatism, trust, and common interest (especially after they have learned a good deal about each other)—but they also work hard to retain their unique culture (see Figure 4.1).

In a pluralistic social environment, although group A and group B each retain their uniqueness, they are persuaded that they both benefit from cooperating in a specific area of common interest (the shaded area). The fresh growth that evolves from their joint energies is one of the positive characteristics of a coexistence society. For example, when Spanish-speaking and English-speaking families

FIGURE 4.1. The Dynamics of Coexistence

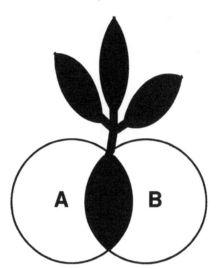

cooperate in working for an improved language program at their grade school, both sides may be enriched culturally, and the children may be able to stage a folk festival at the end of the school year. In such an instance, each group is willing to give up some of its sovereignty in exchange for tangible shared benefits.

Furthermore, coexistence requires that all groups share power and resources rather than let one group accumulate a monopoly. In conflict situations, this type of society is most likely to use mediation, and to attain win/win outcomes that satisfy all parties. In fact, intergroup cooperation generates what Ruth Benedict called "synergy"—outcomes that are greater than a sum of the separate contributions of each participant (Benedict 1970; Harris 1970).

In a coexistence reality, decentralized decision making rises from the grassroots level by means of citizen participation. A coexistence society, by definition, contains no strangers, and again because it respects difference, learns to live with some unpredictability. This approach seems appropriate for a planet full of increasingly pluralistic cities and nations.

## IMPLICATIONS FOR PERSONAL
## AND INTERGROUP CONFLICTS

According to the analysis of five kinds of conflict in Chapter 2, establishment-minority relations are characterized by power imbalance and closed-minded ideologies. Reuse of these two variables helps us clarify why a segregationist approach to ethnic minorities is likely to lead to conflict escalation–while coexistence makes de-escalation more likely.

A range of possible establishment-minority relations is illustrated in Table 4.1.

TABLE 4.1. Types of Establishment-Minority Relations

| Actual Power Arrange-ments | Ideology of Participants | |
|---|---|---|
| | Flexible and Inclusive | Closed and Exclusive |
| No Unit Has a Monopoly (.5 / .5) | 1) COEXISTENCE<br><br>Participation of equals.<br><br>Cooperation based in consensus.<br><br>e.g., Switzerland or Hawaii. | 3) DISAGREEMENT<br><br>Reluctant collabora-tion.<br><br>Compromises within turbulence.<br><br>e.g., South Africa. |
| One Unit Has a Monopoly (1 / 0) | 2) INTEGRATION<br><br>The strong attracts the others.<br><br>Accept some loss in favor of greater gains.<br><br>e.g., U.S.A. | 4) SEGREGATION<br><br>Submission based on coercion.<br><br>Clash normatively or violently.<br><br>e.g., The Kurds in Turkey |

Again, five outcomes become viable:

1. Inclusiveness and power balance tend to produce an environment of trust, cooperation, and consensus. After full processes of questioning, debating, arguing, or voting, the outcome is considered worthwhile by all parties. Conflict is minimized,

and specific conflicts tend to be settled amicably in a win/win manner. Similarly, this is the social environment in which *coexistence* becomes feasible. The working together of diverse language-culture cantons in Switzerland or racial groups in Hawaii serve as pragmatic examples of this option.

2. An open ideology and power monopoly create a situation in which the strong party persuades the others to accept *integration* (by its standards). When such a policy prevails, the weaker parties take comfort in knowing that although they face a short-term lose/win option, becoming like the establishment has some long-term advantages. The issue of integration is particularly relevant when large groups of refugees or immigrants have to be absorbed with minimum disruption to the host population (as was typical of Irish, Italian, and Jewish immigrant groups in the United States during the late nineteenth century, and of Jews into Israel since 1950).

3. When all parties have similar power capacities, a closed ideology creates the turbulence of value-based *disagreement*—especially during times of rapid social change. Thus, in South Africa some white conservatives were very upset about the dismantling of apartheid, and some black tribes, though they have been victimized by whites, were still preoccupied with violently settling intertribal scores. However, former rivals or enemies (such as the African National Congress and the white South African government) showed a reluctant readiness for compromises. They did so because they do not have enough power to obtain a more favorable outcome, and perhaps in order to avoid escalating the disagreements into mutually destructive (lose/lose) violence.

4. Closed ideology and power monopoly allow the strong to practice *segregation*—i.e., to oppress and victimize their weak populations in the classic win/lose manner. This situation was typical of black-white relations in the United States before the Martin Luther King era, and is still typical of many other countries in Africa, Europe, and Asia.

5. However, outright *violence* (e.g., Kurd-Turk relations in the Middle East during 1991-1992) suggests that if the weaker party refuses to submit, the cost of maintaining conformity

escalates. In fact, the outcome may well become a vicious cycle of violent rebellion and backlash. In such cases, both sides, and the environment, pay heavily.

## SUMMARY

This chapter has looked at some connections between institution-alized societal arrangements and conflict. Segregationist societies are rife with conflicts despite their efforts to settle disagreements in authoritarian ways. In integrationist societies, if the minority groups are willing to undergo a partial deculturation, conflict is less intense. Ability to live with short-term compromises may well lead to long periods of peace (as is characteristic of the past few hundred years of Scandinavian history).

Despite the difficulties of transition to a coexistence kind of soci-ety (as illustrated by the agonies that the European Common Market countries are undergoing at the end of this century), such a society may well promise a decreasingly conflictual future.

## CODA

It seems appropriate to conclude this chapter with an excerpt from a short article written by Robert Fulghum (1987):

Most of what I really need to know about how to live, and how to be, I learned in kindergarten. . . . Share. Play fair. Don't hit people. Put things back where you found them. Clean up your own mess. Don't take things that aren't yours. Say you're sorry when you hurt somebody. . . . Live a balanced life. . . . When you go out into the world, watch for traffic, hold hands and stick together. Be aware of wonder. . . . Think what a better world it would be if . . . as nations, we had a basic policy of always putting things back where we found them and cleaning up our own messes. And it is still true, no matter how old you are, when you go out into the world, it is best to hold hands and stick together.

Chapter 5

# Conflicts Generated by Victimization

## VICTIM BEHAVIORS IN MODERN SOCIETY

The twentieth century is noted for its high levels of violence. The news media and learned studies seem full of reports about world-wide and regional wars, stereotypic condemnation (if not outright genocide) of whole peoples, stock-market swindles of consumer groups or small investors, civil strife between tribes or ethnic populations, women and/or children abused by violent men, upset (often enraged) men who climb towers or enter public buildings and shoot anyone in sight, sophisticated forms of urban violence practiced by local police, or teenage pupils bringing loaded revolvers to school. Each of these produces its crop of involuntary deprivation, suffering, loss, frustration, and anger–both among the direct victims and among their survivors.

Actually, the concept "victim" has several interrelated meanings. In contemporary English, as in Biblical Hebrew, the word connotes the sacrificial offering of a plant, animal, or human being as part of a religious ceremony. Worshipers felt the need to destroy or kill (i.e., to victimize) someone or something in order to feel closer to, or to appease, a deity.

The idea of victim has since been redefined to indicate a person and/or group who have been:

1. involved in a natural disaster, in a human-caused accident (or who seem accident prone);
2. deprived of something important through no fault of their own (e.g., the family of a soldier listed as missing);
3. dominated or oppressed by others who are more powerful; or

4. hurt intentionally (e.g., blacks in the apartheid system of South Africa, women who have been raped, pensioners who have been robbed) or unintentionally (e.g., neighbors deprived of their homes through urban renewal, or persons contaminated by nuclear wastes dumped in their environment).

In this chapter, the focus is on people who suffer repeated deliberate traumatic stress (Baden 1991; Halevi 1992; Hareven 1983).

Montville (1987) has summarized some common components of being victimized. The victim is at first stunned by some violent act that shatters a previous norm or equilibrium. As with the Jews or the gypsies in Nazi Germany, one's identity or affiliation with an ethnic/historic group (seen by many as a basic need of all human beings) is turned suddenly and arbitrarily into a liability. When victims are convinced that they have been attacked undeservedly, feelings of loss may be accompanied by anger, and anger may grow into rage. Victims may also become fearful of unpredictable future attacks—often intensified by feeling powerless to provide for their own safety. Such a combination of suffering, anger, powerlessness, and fear are raw materials for becoming closed and defensive.

No healthy person or group enjoys being the target of bigotry or violence. If a threat of repeated violation persists, victim groups tend to become closed and fanatic, to polarize the world into a "we vs. them" battleground, and to turn to violence—in turn becoming victimizers of others. Some victims respond by internalizing their feelings and behaving passively, but in others, the desire for vengeance or financial restitution can become an all-consuming obsession (Cohen 1990).

## FOUR TYPES OF VICTIMS

How victimization may destroy previously adequate ways of coping is elaborated in the next section's discussion of crisis theory. It is enough for us to recognize that repeated arbitrary traumas often turn those who experience them into victims. In fact, there are four types of victims:

## Those Who Become Vulnerable

One type of victim includes people or groups who have been made vulnerable by the experience (e.g., the "Uncle Tom," or the passive child repeatedly beaten by her violent father). As emotionally disabled persons suffering from learned helplessness, they expect additional disasters, suppress or deny their feelings, become immobilized, or suffer a chronic lack of self-respect. If they belong to a stigmatized ingroup and cannot leave it because of outgroup coercion, they may become infected with self-hatred (Lewin 1948; Rothman 1965). They may try to keep a low profile, pass themselves off as members of the majority group, or feel afraid, ashamed, guilty, or depressed. They may also utilize their minority status as an excuse for not taking risks, or for escaping responsibility for their own lack of progress (Seligman 1975).

The persistence of such victim behaviors is well illustrated by a humorous "Dry Bones" cartoon from the September 1, 1982 *Jerusalem Post* newspaper. It shows two men in a continuing friendly conversation. One of them recites Israel's many successes of that time: the peace treaty with Egypt, the successful blowing up of Iraq's nuclear plant, the driving of terrorists out of Beirut, and the country's standing up to world pressures. His partner replies that all these wonderful events make him nervous, because he misses "his Jewish insecurity."

## Those Who Stifle Anger

Close to the above but less obvious is another type of victim—minorities or peoples who have been subjugated for a long time. They do not lack self-respect. However, being low in hope, they lose their initiative and seem apathetic (Humphrey 1981; Montville 1989b), especially when they see no way to remedy the situation or to leave their group of origin. The longer their subjugation lasts, the more likely they are to be stifling a growing anger. The Palestinians before the Intifada or the blacks in South Africa after years of apartheid serve as examples of this category.

### Those Who Express Rage

Unlike those who internalize or repress their anger, the third type of victim externalizes feelings. Full of outrage at the injustice of their condition, they may hate the majority that oppresses them, insist that their suffering never be forgotten, disturb the status quo by violating norms, and/or demand special consideration. In extreme cases, they resort to violence and terror. Their rage, turned into hatred, may be passed on from generation to generation—as is characteristic of some Appalachian families (in the United States) or Serbs and Croats in former Yugoslavia. They are often motivated by a powerful need to avenge their personal pain and humiliation or those of their group (Grier and Cobbs 1968; Dimsdale 1980).

### Those Who Survive Constructively

A fourth type is represented in victims who have survived the ordeal, found ways to heal themselves, do not hate or blame the victimizer, and have no need to revenge themselves on members of their own family or of other groups. They retain or have regained a constructive normal lifestyle, and can be found volunteering to help others to do the same. Japanese survivors of the atom bombing of Hiroshima, just as many Jewish survivors of the Holocaust, provide examples of this fourth category.

## A CASE EXAMPLE: A VICTIMIZED REFUGEE
## BECOMES FREE

The autobiographical case history that follows illustrates the fourth kind of victim mentioned above. This is the story of a victim who suffered, survived, became rehabilitated, and was able to return to normal living. In her own words, beginning in 1976:

> the war for the control of the high-rise hotel in Beirut was underway. The Holiday Inn, a sniper's nest until it was burned out, was two blocks away from my apartment. Heavily armed militia roamed our street. Pack the bags, bundle up the chil-

dren, and travel for safety to Amman. . . . In Amman I was greeted by my sobbing Aunt A. Refugees again? Our generation and now yours? When will it end?

Unlike the previous generation of Palestinians, we did go back to Beirut. As the situation intensified, however, we left again, this time for London . . . when my mother called . . . to tell me excitedly that "Pnina" had just called her and was coming to visit. . . . My mother loved Pnina but in my hot angry, youthful days I resented this woman, this Jew. She had stayed in Palestine because she was Jewish while my family and I had to be supported and exiled. . . . I could not deal with the fact that there I was, loving and admiring a Jewish woman! My enemy!

1982: The Israelis invaded Lebanon. Bombardment, siege, and evacuation. . . . The massacres. The fear. The whole insecurity of being a Palestinian again. . . . One can uproot from a place but not from one's skin, one's history, one's people. The dilemmas. The sense that we had betrayed those we left behind. . . . The sense of helplessness and total incapacitation, of loss, and that immense guilt.

Sitting . . . in the safety of my suburban American home, missing my parents, friends, and way of life, out of touch with my culture and my roots, I cried for having lived 40 years over which I had absolutely no control. . . . I took up my pen and wrote "Dear Leah," addressing an imaginary Jewish woman . . . (asking) her when it would be over for both of us. That letter, written in utter despair, became the epilogue of a novel, my first. . . . Writing was the best therapy for me, as I aired all of my anger . . . over the Palestinian tragedy.

1987: I was asked to read the "Dear Leah" letter, and share a stage with another Palestinian writer . . . and two Israelis. . . . Having accepted, I could not then imagine going to the preconference dinner and sharing bread with my enemies. I . . . had been preaching tolerance and understanding, I had stated my views in non-erasable print. I . . . went and found commonalities which surprised me. The wall between me and anything Jewish or Israeli started to crumble. From then on it was easier to participate in dialoguing with the enemy.

November 31, 1987: I flew to London. My father had passed away unexpectedly. Another Palestinian being buried, in exile, away from his Jerusalem. My hatred . . . and grief comingled into a crescendo that belied all recent acceptance of peaceful coexistence. People would be coming. . . . I went over to my neighbour, then I asked to borrow some of her chairs. We stood and cried together as she told me how she had been living with death all of her life. She had lost two brothers . . . to the Nazi Holocaust.

December 9, 1987: The Intifada. A resurgence of hope, pride and dignity. The Palestinians had taken their destiny into their own hands. . . . Yes, we can talk now. Yes, we were paying the price of freedom with the blood of our children. Yes, we have earned our place at the negotiating table. It was a tremendous feeling.

February 1990: I took part in a dialogue conference with American-Palestinian and American-Jewish women. It presented many dilemmas. . . . When I saw one of the American-Jewish women fighting a battle within herself during the conference . . . wanting to be objective yet afraid to betray her people by doing so, I was reminded of myself. I could see deep into her very heart, into recesses of her soul where she, herself, had not yet dared to look. I saw a Leah, respecting her Palestinian counterpart as they both extended, though fearfully, their hands in peace. (Jabour 1993)

## *SOME COMPONENTS OF VICTIM BEHAVIOR*

We may enhance our understanding of the forces that combine to create and preserve the victimized person or group by studying Figure 5.1.

When fear, ignorance, and anger combine in various ways, the outcomes might be hatred, efforts to humiliate, and efforts to victimize others. When all three variables overlap in a person or a group, the outcome is likely to be fanaticism.

We can understand how victims, just as the writer of the above case history, grieve for loss, are hurt, and begin to hate those who have victimized them. At first, the Palestinian writer saw all Jews

Figure 5.1. Three Components of Close-Mindedness

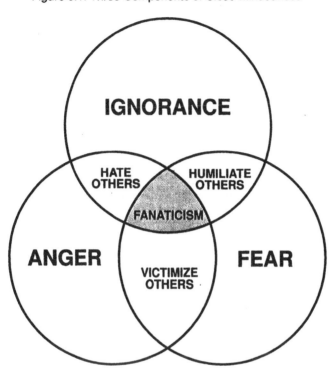

(not just Israelis) as the enemy of her people. In the initial stages, she suffered from a powerful closedness, expressed in a sense of righteousness. However, this woman's fear regarding an unpredictable future did not stop her from taking risks. She published articles and books, met (reluctantly) with Jewish women, and became empathic to the suffering of the other side. Anger at years of arbitrary exclusion, insults, and exploitation caused her to retain a stereotype of the other group, but pride in her people's Intifada and the therapy of writing helped her outgrow them. She was even surprised by her own feelings of understanding and love for specific Jewish women she encountered (Susser 1992). She did not succumb to ignorance, which could have worsened her victim's sense of disconnectedness. Perhaps because her mind and soul remained open and observant, she emerged from victimization and became free from its constraints.

Since victimization often destroys previously adequate ways of coping, crisis theory can help us understand some of its negative dynamics. Resiliant people or systems in crisis may be temporarily incapable of coping with some unexpected, grievous loss, or an external event such as a train wreck, flood, or being taken hostage. But, over a relatively short time period, normal human systems in crisis can experience both mourning and healing. However, when victims are highly vulnerable, or the situation is one of repeated and arbitrary shocks, an initial crisis reaction may turn into a serious pathological condition that, as mentioned above, may be passed on from generation to generation (Charney 1990; Viano 1990).

In continuation of the four hypotheses posed in Chapter 2, we might consider a fifth one–the less one or both sides in a serious conflict have been victimized, the lower the probability that the conflict will escalate into violence.

## THE VICTIM AS A CULTURAL ARCHETYPE

According to the psychiatrist Karl Jung, the term "archetype" describes a type of human behavior that has been known for many generations and in many cultures. Some examples of archetypes include: the matriarch, the villain, the great hero, the traitor (Norway's World War II leader Quisling is a modern equivalent), the wise elder, or the victim. Such archetypes often guide our day-to-day behavior. According to Jung, they become part of one's personality as a result of normal socialization. The ideas, implanted as they are from our earliest years, permeate our definition of human nature and determine how we understand the meaning of behaviors and events.

For example, from the time of the Roman conquest of Israel until the Holocaust of the twentieth century, many Jews have internalized a self-image of the victimized people. These Jews make intense efforts not to forget the horrors of the Holocaust, and not to allow others to forget it. They may want to expel all Palestinians from the Jewish state, and do not believe the promises of gentiles guaranteeing Israel's borders. In fact, they may get caught up in a fundamental certainty that the whole world is against them. One-sided press coverage of events in Israel feeds into this sense of victimization, and even strengthens it (Chetkow-Yanoov 1985; Cohen 1990).

Similarly, the Palestinians, remembering the golden past of Arab culture and longing for their former homes in what has become Israel, protest the present reality, which only humiliates them. Having also internalized the self-image of victim, Palestinians do not accept a definition of the West Bank and Gaza as territories conquered by the Jews in a defensive war, do not believe the promises of the Jews, and make efforts not to forget (or let others forget) the atrocities which they have suffered (Knudsen-Hoffman 1993; Shipler 1986).

For about 100 years, both the Jewish-Israeli and the Palestinian peoples found themselves stuck in a dead-end situation. They both return repeatedly to what they learned in the past—to the role of the suffering victim in a hostile or uncertain environment. Like a videotape repeated over and over, each side continued to distrust, to hate, and to blame the other for its current and continuing plight. If playing out a deep-rooted victim role has become a source of secure identity for individuals or for a group, each subsequent generation will be socialized to repeat it. In fact, any suggestion that they change this behavior may be perceived as a threat to both their identity and their survival.*

## *VICTIMIZERS*

Victimizers of today are likely to have been victims earlier in their lives (Dimsdale 1980). Victimizers typically seek scapegoats among persons or groups weaker than themselves—as a way of coping with whatever they find frightening or infuriating.** Their targets are

---

*This argument can explain why small but vocal groups of Palestinian and Jewish fundamentalists are absolutely against the success of the September 1993 peace agreement between the PLO and Israel. They cannot support the agreement unless they find new ways to satisfy their basic human and group needs.

**Over the centuries, demagogues have played on fear and anger reactions in large population groups to separate peoples, to distract attention from shortcomings, and to consolidate power. The topic is not elaborated on in this book.

usually persons or groups who are not organized for self-defense (Kelman and Hamilton 1989; Miller 1986).

Behaving in predictable ways, victimizers may:

1. take money or property by fraud, or by threatening dire consequences if they are resisted;
2. deny basic rights to members of minority or inferior groups;
3. hate their victims and emphasize their unreliability (i.e., that they are to be watched carefully);
4. find justification for engaging in slander, discrimination, oppression, and exploitation; and
5. use violence, often killing those who are defined as inferior.

The longer people function as victims or as victimizers, the more likely they are to appear like each other. Very often, when victims "graduate" from the weaker to the stronger side, they repeat the same pattern (e.g., the former slave who becomes a vicious emperor, African leaders who exploit their own group mercilessly, or the beaten child who becomes an abusive parent). Whatever the outcome, they often appear to survive in a painful dance for two—having become dependent on each other for their identity and survival (Danieli 1985; Silverman 1975).

## VICTIMIZATION MAKES CONFLICTS CONTINUE

In any continuing conflict situation, we might well speculate about what normal and/or pathological needs are being satisfied for the humiliated and the humiliator, for the conquered and the conqueror, the stigmatized and the powerful, the constant loser and the confident winner, the exploited and the exploiter (see Chapter 3).

Given, however, that successful conflict resolution includes recognition of the needs of the opponent and a willingness to compromise, victims are unable to do this if their own basic human needs, say, for identity or security, have been negated by a powerful establishment (Harkabi 1972; Volkan 1988). Just as they have been dehumanized, victims are likely to dehumanize other groups.

Warren (1987) suggests that many such victims suffer from "conflict neurosis," which includes:

1. blaming the other side for all these troubles ("they are immoral and unreliable");
2. dwelling on personal and peripheral issues rather than central ones;
3. not trusting anyone who does not condemn the opponent; and
4. twisting facts or oversimplifying history, in order to support the victim's viewpoint or position.

Living as they often do in a starkly dichotomized world, victims may not only be certain that everyone else is against them, but all persons on the other side are also stereotyped as uncaring, hostile, and untrustworthy.

Rather than trying to settle long-standing conflicts, some victims vent their frustration and rage on members of the majority group. When the aggressor is too dangerous (a strong target may lash back effectively or shame them publicly), they can feel important by abusing some scapegoat who is weaker than themselves—often including peripheral members of their own (Palestinian or black South African) people. Thus, many victims become victimizers, and the vicious circle continues.

Morally alienated, insecure, full of resentment, and/or ill with self-hatred, victims may become paranoid enough to feel justified to strike first, before any enemy tries to hurt them. Also, as the Serbs in Yugoslavia, the Armenians in Turkey-Iraq, or rival black tribes in Liberia, their own past suffering does not stop them from victimizing others (Charney 1990). Rather, they seem programmed to repeat what others have done to them. Not only are many victims ready to eliminate real or imagined opposition by violent means, they may justify immoral behaviors (e.g., telephone-tapping or car-bombing) as essential for their survival. With such a worldview, formerly exploited colonial peoples, or children beaten by violent parents, are likely to be in the center of ongoing or later conflicts, and not among those who try to resolve them (Harkabi 1972; Montville 1989a; Volkan 1988).

## *SUMMARY*

This chapter introduced four types of long-victimized individuals, groups, and even large ethnic populations, as well as to the behavioral patterns typical of victimizers. All such systems seem driven by fear and anger. Because both victims and victimizers are consumed with unmet needs (often trying to satisfy their needs in antisocial ways), they seem to play a central role in ongoing or escalating conflicts. Like all victims in all parts of the world, they seem to repeat the only pattern of behavior with which they are familiar.

We would do well to focus on the urgency of finding new ways to resolve conflicts among victimized ethnic groups. When rage and fear are prevalent, routine negotiations and cease-fire arrangements (as in Bosnia during 1993-1995) become ineffective. One fresh model for breaking out of this behavioral pattern is presented in Chapter 6.

# PART III:
# SOCIAL WAYS TO COPE
# WITH CONFLICTS

Chapter 6

# Some Basic Ways to Practice Conflict Resolution

## *INTRODUCTION*

In Chapter 5, we came to the conclusion that victimized persons and population groups can be so damaged that they become central in long-persisting conflicts and in conflicts that escalate into high levels of violence. Thus, if we hope to cope effectively with conflicts generated by the victimization, we should not be tempted into blaming the victims (for example, abused wives or enraged African Americans in Los Angeles) for their condition, nor may we ask them to solve the problem solely by modifying their behavior (Davis and Hagen 1992). Second, we have to consider the possibility that some types of victims are not helpable. Just as the Israelites in the Exodus who longed to return to the fleshpots of Egyptian slavery, some victims are destroyed by their experience. The Israelites had to wander in the desert until that generation died out.

On the other hand, when I, an obvious American, spent two weeks in Hiroshima (in August 1986), I did not encounter anger against Americans. Not knowing a word of their language, I was totally dependent on local people to find my way around. Japanese women and men of all ages helped me cheerfully (seemingly well beyond their norms of politeness) throughout my stay in their midst. If they retained a residue of hatred (or denial) from their victimization by the atom bombing, I could not detect it. In this connection, it is worth noting how Americans lost their hatred of the Japanese, and for that matter of the Germans, almost immediately after World War II.

Similarly, studies of abused children who grow up to become parents suggest that although one-third of them are abusive to their offspring, the other two-thirds find ways to escape from repeating the pattern (Altemeier et al. 1986; Browne and Finkelhor 1986; Draucker 1992). In Israel, too, about 30 percent of the known Holocaust survivors pass the victim syndrome on to a second generation, but the others do not hate all Germans and seem to be living normal lives. Some are even functioning as lay counselors to other survivor families in a voluntary organization called Amcha.

Durbach (1993) explains the matter succinctly. If Nelson Mandela, "the man the white government jailed for 28 years can put peace above retribution, perhaps–just perhaps–his people, those oppressed by a century of apartheid rule, can do the same." They will also need to find ways to deal with their long-accumulated rage in conciliatory ways, rather than persisting in the current waves of black-on-black violence. The next section of this chapter deals with such issues.

## HOW CAN VICTIMS BE HELPED?*

For reasons outlined in Chapter 5, victimization must be remedied in order to enhance the practice of conflict resolution. Based on current social science knowledge and on principles from the healing professions, ten types of help can be made available to victims:

### Learn To Cope with Fear and Anger

Although both fear and anger serve useful purposes in times of danger or exploitation, victims usually suffer from a glut of these emotions. If they are to break free of the behavioral syndrome outlined in Chapter 5, they must be able to give expression to their pain and hurt–rather than deny them, be ashamed of them, or actually hide them from others (especially from their own children or spouses). It is important that they learn to cope with their fear and rage in healthier ways than they did before. They might first become sensitive to clues of fear-induced reactions in themselves, in order to

---

*It would be interesting, but is beyond the scope of this chapter, to analyze what kind of a parallel but different healing process could be designed to help victimizers stop traumatizing groups that they once hated and exploited.

recognize them immediately and overcome them. They will probably be helped if they can validate their suffering in a supportive group setting.

Instead of personal depression, denial, suspicion, blaming, reactionary conservatism, or humiliating others, they might seek temporary relief in ways described in the section on dealing with continuous tension or pressure (below). One way of coping more adequately is to sublimate one's feelings by channeling energies into social action—to protest some urgent problem or create a voluntary initiative to alleviate it. Battering men may, as an outcome of group experiences, become sufficiently rehabilitated to stop their automatic violent reactions (Parsloe 1987). At such a point, individuals and groups become able to register that others also have needs, and that alternatives to blaming or hitting are effective.*

### Take Steps To Enhance One's Self-Esteem

As in the feminist movement, victims trying to emerge from their exploited minority status may be helped by small group sessions on improved self-image and skills-training in assertiveness (Klein 1992). Some reach a similar outcome through their involvement in psychodrama or community theatre (Alfi 1986; Chetkow-Yanoov 1978; Moreno 1944).

Seen in a community-wide focus, the self-esteem of former victims can be enhanced by taking part in a variety of positive group experiences—such as a special summer day-camp for mothers of large families, the policy-making body of a neighborhood renewal project, a leadership training course for poverty-neighborhood activists, or an intercultural festival of ethnic cooking and folkdancing. It is refreshing to be able to display one's culture and its artifacts proudly (rather than be ashamed of them, as when they were associated with victimhood). A healthy self-image also allows us to

---

*The intervention model proposed here, based as it is on psychiatric theory and practice, has to be expanded so that it can be effective with large population groups. Perhaps we can adapt theatre and television techniques to get the job done relatively quickly. We do not seem to have enough time to do the task on a one-by-one basis.

appreciate the characteristics of other cultures–because our identity no longer depends on someone else being inferior to us.

### Meet with Members of the Victimizer Group

During the healing process, former victims may benefit from a structured encounter meeting with members of those whom they once called the enemy (i.e., whom they perceived as the victimizer). Intense guided contacts and joint activities, although entered reluctantly at first, become a bridge to knowing the other side as human beings rather than as archetypes or stereotyped categories (Hoffman, 1982).

Noncompetitive face-to-face or small group encounters can help the participants ventilate enough to alleviate deeply held fears, and to allow the weak side to behave as an equal. Together, they may be able to learn collaborative problem-solving skills. New friendships bring an end to self-isolation, and make possible the finding of superordinate goals (such as volunteering to help mentally disabled children) that both sides can share. Not only do both sides overcome their group's fear of strangers, but both feel strong enough to answer the cries of "traitor" from the still fearful members of their groups of origin (Chetkow-Yanoov 1985; Zak 1992).

### Reaching the "Enough!" Condition

As with any habitual or addictive behavior, professional helpers must be sensitive to when victimized people or groups have become sufficiently uncomfortable, dissatisfied, or disgusted with themselves to make continuing as usual intolerable. Former victims require a lot of support when they want "to quit" but do not know how. They have to feel ready to stop acting like martyrs, retreating into an exclusive fortress of fundamentalism, demonizing the other side, or attacking those with whom they do not agree.

As is normal to almost all growth experiences, such a desire for change will probably be accompanied by anxiety and fear. However, with professional counseling and lots of peer support, these feelings become sufficiently weakened that they no longer cancel the victims' desire to break away from their former behavior patterns.

## Mourn Giving Up the Victim Self-Image

Within the norms of the prevailing culture, a person or group trying to stop relying on the crutch of victimhood may need to mourn the loss of this crutch. It is extremely difficult to cease a habitual behavior without undergoing a formal parting ceremony or ritual, and experiencing the relief of tears in the presence of others. Only after grieving fully (e.g., for someone who has been part of our life for many years, or for a long-standing victim identity that once helped us to survive) can one let go of the old status–and get on with the business of life by taking the first steps toward reintegration within the new status of widow, nonsmoker, or nonviolent person.

To complete a wholesome mourning process, a former victim may require help from a therapist or a friend who is capable of supplying empathy and emotional support during the difficult post-loss period. It is equally important to work toward increased self-understanding and to learn some skills in conquering one's habits. Here, too, a support group (such as Alcoholics Anonymous) may be helpful. A completed mourning process should end the tendency to self-pity and give former victims new self-respect.

## Cancel All Obligations and No Longer Demand Compensation

In religious parlance, we are told that the victim must forgive the aggressor in order to become free. In other words, the victim willingly gives up the intention of taking revenge and cancels the debts that were formerly claimed as compensation for past humiliations, deprivations, and suffering. It is important to stress that forgiving the victimizer for past wrongs involves a process of continuous learning and reinforcement and has little to do with forgetting what took place in the past (Levin 1992). Some European survivors of Japanese internment camps, for example, claim they did not hate their Japanese overseers (as most victims do). In fact, these survivors contend that they were able to transcend the "eye for an eye" mentality, and that gave them life (Bloom 1990). The act of forgiving also requires the internalization of new hate-free communication skills, such as empathic listening (Cornelius and Faire 1989; Klein 1992; Rosenberg 1983).

If done successfully, this debt cancelling can reopen victims' ability to appreciate others and to get back in harmony with themselves (Stauffer 1987). When former victims can let go (or "call off the war"), they also stop punishing themselves, forgive themselves for their own past mistakes, and drop the fear/guilt/anger/blaming from their repertoire of coping behaviors. It is just like a slave being set free, or the "burden" falling off the shoulders of John Bunyan's pilgrim (Bunyan 1909).

Montville (1987) tells how Mme. Irene Laure, a former member of the French parliament from Marseilles and a victim of Nazi barbarism, changed the atmosphere at a crucial post-World War II conference at Caux (in Switzerland) when she admitted that her hatred of all Germans was wrong, and asked their forgiveness. In a more recent situation, the Palestinian leader Hanna Siniora was able to say: "Each side has a long list of grievances, but they should be consigned to history. Instead of competing for the victim's pride, we must try for a new constructive mood" (Swartz 1987).

In the same way, someone with appropriate skills (see discussion of the "healer" role, below) might help former victimizers to admit publicly that injustice has been done, repent, and apologize for their past actions (Charney 1990; Kelman 1991; Montville 1993). In 1970, German chancellor Willy Brandt did this symbolically when he kneeled (in Warsaw) before the Polish memorial to victims of World War II. In 1991 President Lech Walensa of Poland visited Israel and made a clear public apology for the Polish cooperation with the Nazis against the Jews during World War II. We can only speculate about what would happen if similar apologies were uttered in other conflictual situations—between Japanese war heroes and former Korean prisoners, between Singhalese and Tamils, Hindus and Moslems (in India), or Jewish Israelis and the Palestinians.

Israel's Druse and Bedouin Arabs still resort to a formalized *sulcha* (forgiveness) ceremony to settle interclan feuds. When a member of one family has been injured or killed by someone from another clan, the traditional pattern of redeeming the family's honor with revenge can be stopped by declaring a sulcha. This creates a binding cease-fire for a few days, during which local and regional notables form a reconciliation committee and activate a process of interfamily mediation. A settlement often involves the paying of compensation to the injured party, and once this has been accepted, the need to redeem the family/tribal honor is cancelled.

### Undergoing a Symbolic Transformation

The process of healing is much enhanced if victims can be helped to transmute negative historical experiences into something symbolizing a new kind of positive. After hundreds of years of slavery, the Jews who exited from ancient Egypt celebrated Passover as the festival of freedom. Similarly, the death of Jesus of Nazareth took on new meaning in the symbolism of the Resurrection. In the United States of the 1960s, Negroes who had been slaves became proud African Americans when they agreed that "black is beautiful."

### Taking Risks and Making Decisions

Part of the emancipation of former victims is for them to stop blaming everything on others—and to resume taking responsibility for their own decisions and actions. Instead of rationalizing their lack of action or immoral deeds (while seeking vengeance), they should be helped to break free from long-continuing hatred—by means of a completed process of mourning and forgiveness. With sufficient support and opportunities for simulated practice, they can begin to trust themselves, to take small risks, to make choices among real alternatives, or to venture into specific actions which they feared in the past.

The place of decision making in the rehabilitation process is illustrated in Figure 6.1. For example, a battered wife can be encouraged to dare to go to court for a divorce, a widow from a support group might gradually begin to date again, or a well-challenged gang leader might choose to go back to school. During the rehabilitation process, the self-awareness and self-image of these ex-victims is helped to improve. Further, as ex-victimizers begin to trust others in specific situations, they may be able to undertake some highly structured cooperative activity with those whom they once called enemies. With sophisticated staff inputs, they can discover each other's humanity rather than continue to rely on old negative stereotypes/generalizations. Now their slogan may well become: "Let there be change, and let it begin with me."

FIGURE 6.1. The Victim-Rehabilitation Process

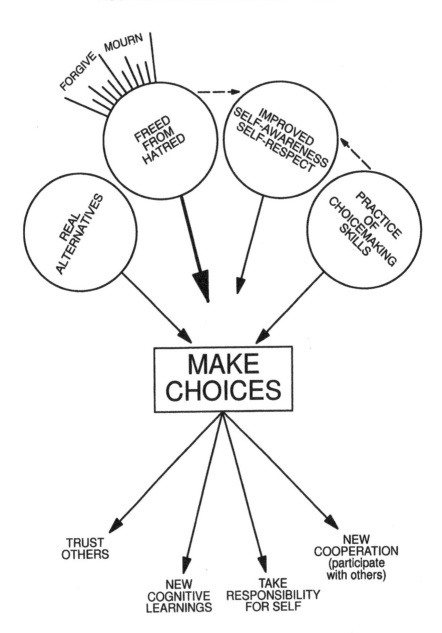

## Convert the Former Negative Interdependence into Partnership

If we can agree that the victim and the victimizer in fact need each other in order to survive, the nature of their relationship must change basically. Once the one has repented and/or the other has forgiven, they can call off their former fight and devote the energy thus freed to living again. They may become sufficiently free to continue interacting—but on a partnership rather than conflictual basis. Now they can pursue and implement superordinate goals together, as equals. One such goal might be to plan an amicable family vacation (with the children) together.

Further, some types of abusive husbands can be rehabilitated by means of a court-mandated therapeutic group experience (Parsloe 1987). When the rehabilitation proceeds well, the men become able to recognize and stop their former habits of violence, but they discover that their wives are becoming confused regarding their less and less violent home behaviors. At this point, they may request parallel group sessions for their wives. When they and their wives experience a joint final session, the rehabilitation is well underway.

On a national level, a postconflict goal might be the pursuit of regional peace among former enemies—as President Sadat of Egypt was able to initiate with Israel in 1977. Since neither the Jewish Israelis nor the Palestinians can make the Middle East flourish alone, if they find a way to become reconciled, perhaps they could manage their scarce natural resources and their holy places on a condominium basis. They could replace the former victim-victimizer (asymmetric) archetype with a new one of peacemakers. In such an eventuality, a form of interdependence continues between them, but it is now based on a high degree of mutuality. Such an outcome could lead to a loose confederation of Middle Eastern states, perhaps along the model of the cantons of Switzerland.

## Functioning Independently

Some victimized persons or groups become so fully healed that they do not need to continue with the former victimizer even in a partnership relationship. When they no longer need to prove how good they are, or to gain respect by exposing the other side's hollowness, they are truly emancipated from the victim role (e.g., a former husband or wife is able, a suitable time after a messy divorce, to enter into a healthy marriage relationship with a new partner).

Such former victims, now free from their early socialization, outgrow or are able to abandon their habit of distrusting, blaming, or hating others. For example, many beaten wives, former addicts, or Holocaust survivors –once rehabilitated or recovered–do "call off the war" with their former victimizers, and can go on to live normal new lives. If they do not forget their former suffering, they can prove superbly empathic to the suffering of others.

## INTERVENTIONS FOR REDUCING CONFLICT ESCALATION

Conflicts should not always be stopped, or, for that matter, prevented. Without friction under our feet, it would be impossible to walk. Lack of an active political opposition is a serious danger to any operational democracy, and under conditions of economic monopoly, customers pay more for the products they consume. Good teachers often create some dissonance in order to make the lesson stimulating.

It may be useful to review John Burton's distinction (1991) between settling disputes and resolving conflicts. Burton contends that dispute settlement takes place in stable authoritarian (i.e., closed) systems, where clashes of interests are negotiated and enforced according to strictly logical norms. When system-wide change is not possible, human groups must accept the rules of those in power or, as in former Balkan and Russian countries in 1992-1993, resort to rebellion and war.

Ideally, the reverse is characteristic of open systems, where the focus is on meeting people's needs and achieving workable compromises. When cooperation is achieved, it is voluntary, and based on all sides gaining something from the process. If conflict resolution is managed well, gradual social change (transformation) takes place without the social environment being torn apart. The emphasis is on doing what is possible to prevent the escalation of normal conflicts into destructive violence, or using participatory processes to de-escalate from violence back into normative conflict behaviors.

If the four components described in Chapter 2 help us to understand conflicts we have experienced, we might profit from examining types of professional intervention that are most appropriate for dealing with each of them (Chandler 1985; Epstein 1970; Pearson and Thoennes 1985). Our goal remains to prevent conflict escalation as much as possible.

### Dealing with Accumulated Tension or Pressure

For example, it is the middle of the Gulf War. Scud missiles are falling on residential parts of Tel Aviv, but Israel's armed forces are not allowed to respond. The population must spend many evening hours in bomb shelters. Everybody is afraid and frustrated, and the situation gets worse as the weeks drag on. What should be done to deal with these widespread feelings?

In situations of ongoing conflict, when a human system cannot close its boundary to tension-making inputs or feedback from its environment, we should first try to bring about some temporary relief. Individually, we might hold unstructured discussions with upset persons, in order to listen and offer empathy for their anxiety, fear, or anger. When their feelings are recognized, people may be able to stop violent attention-getting behaviors, and start listening to each other. We can often produce some catharsis by allowing unrecognized needs, which usually stand behind the powerful feelings mentioned above, to find expression in words or in simple role-play exercises (Green 1990; Rosenberg 1983).

Collectively—during the Gulf War situation, a very warm and human Army spokesman kept the population well-informed by radio and television while they stayed in (gas-proofed) sealed rooms during the Scud attacks. His voice and smile had a universal calming effect. His broadcasts were instrumental in helping the population continue to agree with the policy of nonretaliation.

People who suffer from an accumulation of frustration, fear, and/or anger may also try to retain a modicum of psychological balance by denying that they are upset or that a conflict even exists. It is, therefore, not advisable to start with interventions that might add to their sense of threat or burden. We might rather begin by looking at the problem as they see it, and by showing empathy for their expressed feelings. Later, we can begin gentle questioning, in order to help them face an uncomfortable reality. Even when offering empathy to persons with whom we disagree, it should not be accompanied by argumentation (for example, over the accuracy of specific facts).

Once a person or group can admit that they do have a problem which includes conflict, and that they are not coping well, we can initiate some problem-solving exercises. These should include techniques that facilitate unrestricted thought, self-awareness, and skills-learning. In addition to discussion, people may be helped temporarily to alleviate the emotional stress of conflict by using their muscles. For example, swimming, hitting a punching bag, or running can bring relief by using up some of our nervous energy (see also the suggestions in the next section of this chapter, for helping victims cope specifically with their fear and anger).

Tension may also be eased by means of role-playing (through a symbolic enacting of violence or tears) or through musical and dance activities. We might also help such persons to laugh and relax in a supportive environment of friends and neighbors (Chetkow-Yanoov 1987).

When stress is the product of loss, we might help those affected to complete a process of mourning, or to participate in a ceremony of reconciliation. These activities can help people achieve release from their former "victim" patterns of behavior. Of course, we should make provisions for long-term personal counseling when it is needed.

### Confronting the Closed Person or Group

For example, in a mixed neighborhood of Big City in South Africa, a minority of fanatic white men repeatedly incite all the residents to humiliate and even use violence against the black population in their midst. The white group see themselves as entitled to special privileges, and have no doubt that all other whites or blacks who do not agree with their supremacist views are dangerous or evil. They clash with the police regularly, but never seem to spend any time in jail. How would you penetrate into such a closed group (i.e., cope with their fear/anger/ignorance) in order to cause a change in their behavior?

Joseph Stalin demonstrated one way to stop the activities of veteran revolutionaries (mostly persons of closed personalities)–by executing them. In pluralistic democracies, social norms would sanction our disturbing the equilibrium of such a closed system by enacting and enforcing antiracism legislation (the social control function)–making specific acts of bigotry or incitement punishable. On the other side of the coin, coexistence behaviors, especially if they are new outputs for a formerly closed system, should be clearly rewarded.

As above, in talking with closed persons, listening to their story of suffering with empathy is a prerequisite to initiating any meaningful change. Later, when those involved have advanced beyond denial or fury regarding their condition, or when they have moved from righteous certainty to confusion or self-questioning, they may become more open to an offer of factual information.

Participation in a range of nonthreatening social activities can help create linkages between formerly segregated persons or groups. These could include joint:

1. amateur musical, dance, or theatre groups;
2. attendance at a performance that includes mixed group discussions after the performance;
3. participation in a group to learn a spoken language, handicrafts, carpentry, or flower arrangement;
4. volunteering to help elderly people in their homes, in institutions, or in emergency clinics; or
5. neighborhood improvement activities, especially in racially or culturally mixed environments.

We may be able to lessen the damage of a closed upbringing by exposing all school children routinely to a range of cultures and ethnic groups, and by learning a second language in schools all over our world. We would do well to find ways to open up their system's boundaries and to tempt them with attractive new inputs. New intersystemic linkages, in the form of carefully structured educational encounters with representatives of other groups, are also useful (Rogers 1965).

### To Approximate a Power Balance

For example, in a lower class neighborhood of a middle-size Canadian city, municipal services such as road paving and garbage removal were hardly felt. Despite the many letters and petitions of the residents, the area's lack of prestige and leadership meant that it could be neglected by local bureaucrats and politicians. How would you strengthen the local population sufficiently to force City Hall to pay attention to their legitimate demands for public services?

In situations of power imbalance, the weaker side might need to be empowered by helping it to increase its knowledge, skills, assertiveness, project funding, or access to the news media. The weak might be defended by persons skilled in advocacy who contact the office of the public ombudsman, or initiate an injunction against the mayor in the relevant law court. We might also assist welfare clients to organize themselves into a protest group, or to participate in a multigroup lobby in support of legislative change.

The very strong can be discouraged from abuse of power by calling in the police, exposing their greed in a critical newspaper article, preserving an independent judicial system, bringing a hidden controversy to public attention, and engendering widespread discussion of the underlying issues.

In the Canadian city mentioned in the above example, a community social worker organized a group of about 30 neighborhood residents to attend every open meeting of City Council, to sit in practiced silence through the meeting, and to and clearly write down what they observed and heard. Within three months, Council members were paying attention to the group and the neighborhood's needs. In other words, a sophisticated mixture of resocialization and social control strategies can be used to lessen local power asymmetry—both to strengthen the weaker party and to put limits on the stronger one.

### To Encourage Participatory Decision Making

For example, the slums of Metropolis are constantly disrupted by violent clashes of ethnic gangs. The police believe that they must execute regular raids, and use undercover agents, in order to keep these gangs under control. The minority groups of the region are excluded from all decision-making forums, and the violence seems to be escalating. What would you suggest be done?

In any situation, sustained conflict activities require a large amount of power or resources. Top leadership often engages in bluff, manipulation, and confrontation activities in order to divide the opposition or to overcome it as quickly as possible. Information and communication inputs are deliberately limited or distorted. Democratic processes are short-circuited by means of administrative directives (Warren and Hyman 1966). On the other hand, cooperative activities require much time and maximum participation among power equals. Both full developmental processes and open communication are essential for achieving consensus and group cohesion.

In order to move from an authoritarian style of controlling other persons or systems to a more participatory form of conflict resolution, a number of actions might be tried. For example, we might invite leaders of rival gangs to a prestigious one-day workshop on methods of problem solving. Through role-playing and exercises, the leaders can be helped to experience a process of solving problems without dominating or competing, and gradually become familiar with such conflict resolution strategies as mediation, bargaining, and compromise–in supportive peer settings. In a similar way, they can be taught to play a simulation game that illustrates the costs of unrestricted competition as well as the satisfactions of finding answers to problems through joint effort.

A slightly different approach was tried at the December 1985 annual meeting of the International Center for Peace in the Middle East. The organization staged a simulated international peace conference. During a period of five hours, Jewish members of Knesset, mayors of Arab towns, news media editors, social scientists, and invited experts from abroad played well-orchestrated roles of conference delegates. They experienced the challenge of engaging in hard bargaining and were able to come up with compromise proposals quite different from their initial stands.

When, in treatment, a social worker makes a contract with a client, the client is transformed from a dependent help-seeker into a partner in the healing process. Similarly, people in crisis may be helped by membership in a support group, and violent husbands can be helped to change by participating in a therapeutic group experience (Getzel 1988). Neighborhood volunteers have learned to function in steering committees of urban renewal projects, as parents do on the boards of cooperative nursery schools. Formal structures such as neighborhood associations, food-purchasing cooperatives, municipal committees, federations, or coalitions can also help develop participatory decision-making habits.

Participatory or collaborative strategies include being open to new ideas, providing information to all parties, enhancing open communications, stressing intergroup common interests, creating opportunities for horizontal interaction or networking, engaging in necessary processes of mediation or bargaining, encouraging informal contacts across boundaries, and demonstrating to participants that cooperation is worthwhile. That such matters can be taught to grassroots citizens, school children, community leaders, professionals, and top administrators is demonstrated by the success of the Neighborhood Justice System in San Francisco (described more fully in Chapter 9).

## TAKING ACTION
## AGAINST STRUCTURAL CONFLICTS

Some types of conflict seem to emerge from the very social structures of a stable society (for example, in the vested interests of the communications media, the pragmatism of political leaders, the selfishness of business-industry cartels, or racist policies of service bureaucracies) rather than from interunit rivalries. In conflict situations, the power of such massive opponents is difficult to oppose. When they are both strong and closed-minded, they strive to win their way rather than work to resolve a conflict. In such a situation, we may be forced to function in a confrontational mode in order to achieve structural change. Again, a range of alternative action stances seem possible:

### Preserve the Status Quo

Preserving the status quo usually goes along with conservatism and a reliance on paternalistic bureaucracies. When other participants object to preserving the current situation, the price of keeping order escalates from year to year (as in Chechnya or in South Timor). If some group or faction feels driven to clashing openly with the establishment, the ensuing disorder may cause everyone to lose, and the community is likely to falter.

## *Make Small Adjustments*

Making minor or one-time adjustments actually protects the existing system, or minimizes its need to change (essentials of a conservative environment). It does give birth to a small degree of reluctant nonincremental change. The side richest in resources (for example, the local establishment) might try to persuade weaker partners (such as a neighborhood recreation center) to accept its definition of required changes. Even though the weaker side may lose totally, it cannot remain silent. Perhaps it is better to have protested and lost rather than not to have protested at all.

## *Promote Incremental Changes*

Incremental changes are usually the outcome of an innovative thrust. A specific citizen initiative for a conflict management or peer-mediation program for fourth grade pupils in an impoverished neighborhood of San Francisco did lead to additive improvements in the situation (Chetkow-Yanoov 1984 and 1985; Davis 1983). When meaningful change is too frightening, players may have to compromise on small changes, or wait for more promising future opportunities. In this manner, public interest lobbyists try to bring about needed alterations in existing legislation or prevent the enactment of laws they consider undesirable.

## *Undergo a Transformation*

Conflicts can be transformed if the participating organizations or the community are open to accepting change and taking risks (Warren 1965). Such conditions enable the parties to attain together (often with skilled third-party assistance) something that no one could achieve alone. For example, in one city, after a three-year process of deliberate gestation, domestic conflicts and divorce proceedings were handled by a new mediation/counseling service instead of being routed through a standard adversary (court) process. The situation had been transformed.

## *IMPLICATIONS*

This chapter has focused on matching professional intervention with the type of conflict situations described in earlier chapters of this book. In particular, professionals will want to know how to alleviate the distress generated by long-lasting conflicts, how to open up a system that is closed, how to create a rebalancing of power or resources among the contenders, and how to encourage a participatory form of decision making.

Professional conflict resolvers must feel comfortable not only with conflicts among individual participants but also with organizational and environmental structures which themselves generate conflicts, and with strategies for helping victims break free from their repetitive behavior patterns. A range of professional roles appropriate for such conflict resolution efforts are presented in the next chapter.

Chapter 7

# Professional Roles in Conflict Resolution

## *INTRODUCTION*

Chapter 6 introduced us to a variety of conflict resolution interventions (e.g., bringing about a balance of power, opening up a closed system, easing tension, rehabilitating former victims, or dealing with institutional racism). We were exposed to conflict situations in which the parties, unable to resolve matters themselves, required professional third-party assistance.

In this chapter we first review and elaborate the five basic types/ phases of conflict outlined in Chapter 2. We then suggest a range of nine appropriate professional behaviors. Each type of conflict seems to generate a characteristic syndrome of behaviors, thus requiring specific professional interventions if that type is to be de-escalated.

## *ANOTHER LOOK AT THE FIVE CONFLICT ALTERNATIVES*

As a social worker, I have become increasingly convinced of the usefulness of a five-phase model (see Figure 7.1) of types of conflict:

### *Unease or Tension Amidst General Consensus*

Even in an environment of general consensus and the desire to preserve current relations, differences of interest may arise.

*Feelings.* In situations of minimal conflict, one or all the parties feel some tension, doubts, suspicions, or mild unease. Former feel-

FIGURE 7.1. A Range of Professional Roles in Conflict Resolution

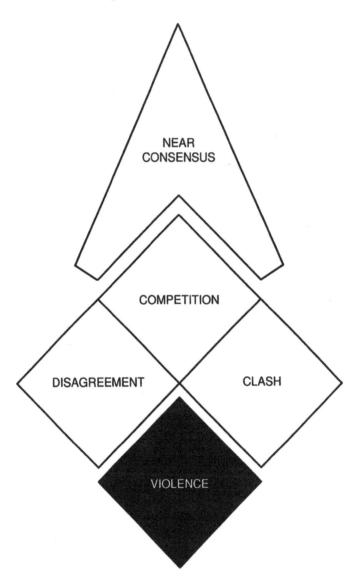

ings of trust may be shaken temporarily. Participants remain certain that the conflict (or its underlying problem) can be managed through dialogue and other forms of interaction. The sides believe in the effectiveness of including all relevant parties in a participatory process.

*Communication.* Open, two-way, and direct communication must continue–especially in situations not connected to the tensions or suspicions that have arisen.

*Power utilization.* When it is relevant to resolving the conflict, power is shared.

*Tactics.* Participants are able to take responsibility for their own part in creating the tension/unease that has arisen. Existing knowledge, attitudes, skills, and habits are seen as adequate for resolving the conflict. The situation receives immediate attention. Even though the parties may raise questions, argue, ask for discussion, debate, or insist on a public vote, they are prepared to cope with the situation cooperatively.

*Expected outcome.* All parties expect to benefit from a win/win outcome.

*Focal Professional Roles.* In minimal conflict situations, the parties must devote time to dialogue until they reach consensus, and are able to implement cooperative ventures typical of the win/win scenario. This implies open and friendly communication channels, much two-way feedback or sharing, and enough optimism and trust to be willing to explore new options. Parties are able to negotiate directly in order for everyone to get what they need or want (Cornelius and Faire 1989; Miedzinski 1992). In this type of environment, third-party intervenors, if they are involved at all, will play a nondirective role such as *facilitator* (which is elaborated later on in this chapter). In the literature, this role is also called stimulator or guide (Ross and Lappin 1967; Rothman 1974).

*Observations.* Most conflicts are resolved at this level. In fact, they may not even be recognized as conflicts. An ideal example of this type of interaction is the method of handling tensions or problems by consensus at Quaker Meetings.

## Contest or Competition

One or all parties involved may seek allies in order to become stronger. These efforts are likely to escalate healthy competition into cutthroat (but still normative) efforts to beat the adversary (see "Clash or Fight" later in this chapter).

*Feelings.* Rivals distrust each other, especially as they contemplate the cost and humiliation of losing. They may feel resentment and anger, especially if they experience repeated losses. One or all parties in the dispute may resort to blaming the other side for the discomfort/inconvenience that has been generated.

*Communication.* Communication lessens significantly, and may be blocked deliberately.

*Power utilization.* The stronger party does everything necessary in order to win. However, today's winner, if not in top form, may become tomorrow's loser.

*Tactics.* The competitors may resort to deliberate confrontation. They may resort to boycotting or challenging (often a bluff) in order to win.

*Expected outcome.* In truly open competitions, some win and others lose. The losers usually yield gracefully, knowing that if they return "in better shape," they might win at another competition. In other words, today's losers admit their shortcomings and go along with the consequences of losing—this time. Since they may win sometimes, they seldom feel victimized, and being temporarily powerless usually does not produce a desire to block other participants or to break the rules. Democratic elections, the Olympic competitions, and agencies that must compete for their allocation of scarce water resources or of philanthropic funds exemplify this type of reality.

*Focal Professional Roles.* In conflicts based on open/fair competition, the role of *expert* or *consultant-educator* is appropriate. This role is effective when the power imbalance is small, and when all participants agree about the usefulness of resolving a conflict.

*Observations.* Although we have seen the advent of noncompetitive games in the last decade, this type of conflict remains typical of relations in most business activities and sports leagues.

### Disagreement or Difference

One or all parties recognize that they are involved in conflict. The longer the situation is ignored, the more likely it is to escalate into a disagreement or fight situation. The sides are likely to get caught up in efforts to preserve ideological purity.

*Feelings.* Initial uncertainty has turned into disappointment and even bitterness. All parties are cautious, and take steps to protect themselves. At this level, the other side is thought to be untrustworthy.

*Communication.* Communication begins to falter and is often distorted by the value or ideological beliefs of the parties involved.

*Power utilization.* No party is strong enough, or sufficiently motivated, to challenge the existing status quo.

*Tactics.* The atmosphere of overall "tension amidst consensus" has been replaced by separation of those involved into sides. If a compromise is impossible, one party may try to veto or block all resolution suggestions. The party that feels wronged may withdraw; if its self-image is still positive, it may encourage a stalemate.

*Expected outcome.* All parties may be satisfied if they can negotiate a compromise.

*Focal Professional Roles.* In such situations, rather than risk costly negative outcomes (such as stalemate, losing everything, or alienating a needed coalition partner), both sides are willing to be pragmatic and make concessions. Although nobody is 100 percent satisfied, all participants are certain that they did the best they could, and that the other side is to be respected. The professional roles of *healer* and *mediator* (or enabler) are central in this type of situation. Sometimes a facilitator can also be helpful.

*Observations.* The sides recognize that a conflict exists, and that compromise is advisable. Many decisions in urban or social planning, as well as in the management of political coalitions, are of this nature.

### Clash or (Fair) Fight

When only one party is strong, it operates as a partisan monopoly, and forces the weaker parties to do society's dirty work for minimal recompense. When the clash is between two strong parties who remain convinced of the rightness of their cause, each party tries to coerce the other side to submit. Functioning within community norms and values, the strong are nevertheless highly motivated to win and to stay in control.

*Feelings.* This level of conflict is often accompanied by fear, strong anger, or by hatred based on prejudice. Both sides operate as closed systems. Formerly neutral groups in the community are often forced to take sides.

*Communication.* Communication media are manipulated in order to present one side as just and the other side as evil and selfish. Distortion of communication, based on overattention to sensational or negative items, is common.

*Power utilization.* In democratic settings, all parties use power blatantly, often within a system of checks and balances created to prevent monopolistic outcomes.

*Tactics.* Powerful opponents may decide to use their resources in order to preserve a status quo favorable to their side. They might oppose, disrupt, or deliberately (but nonviolently) violate norms in order to hurt or shame the other side. They might also lobby, boycott, or file a lawsuit.

*Expected outcome.* Although both sides desire to win (the other must, of course, lose), powerful operators may choose to not go all the way, or even to make profitable coalitions with a strong opponent.

*Focal Professional Roles.* Although rules or norms prevail, closed ideologies and a power imbalance usually involve people who are convinced of the rightness of their own goals. Not only does the weaker side lose, it does so repeatedly. A strong establishment stays in control, and the loser has to keep a low profile or even withdraw. In a democratic society, the opposition has an important function to fulfill and may well resort to using the adversary courtroom system. In coercive realities, the weaker side may take on the role of martyr, insist on arbitration, or seek an advocate. The sides still subscribe to an overall goal of resolving their controversy nonviolently. To do so, they may agree to accept the ruling of a judge or an *arbitrator*, and, as in most bankruptcy proceedings, let such a ruling be implemented by a talented *administrator*.

*Observations.* This type of conflict is exemplified by the efforts of England's social-political elite to gain control over the entire country, or by the continuing efforts of a multinational company such as IBM to dominate the computer field all over the world.

### Violence or War

At this level, the sides abandon all pretense of expecting to resolve their conflict, and prefer to destroy or eliminate the other side. If one or both parties feel victimized, they will probably strive to get revenge.

*Feelings.* Actions are based on self-righteousness and/or fanaticism—derived from a combination of fear, rage, and hatred. The parties may find themselves so obsessed with the situation that they are unable to disengage, or to remember the issue over which the dispute originated. Some parties feel that they must retaliate, strike first, or be ready to victimize others who are weak enough not to strike back. These actions are also expected to deter the other side.

*Communication.* Communication seldom goes beyond blaming the other side. The general attitude is that there is no one to talk to.

*Power utilization.* At this level, power is used violently in order to weaken or destroy the enemy. When both sides appear to be equally strong, the combatants may agree to a cease-fire.

*Tactics.* Morality and social norms are suspended, and either side will use whatever verbally or physically violent means they judge necessary in order to defeat the other side.

*Expected outcome.* To win regardless of the costs, and to coerce the other side into accepting the winner's paradigm of reality.

*Focal Professional Roles.* When one or both sides no longer want to become reconciled, but rather intend to injure or destroy those who oppose them, the conflict escalates into a cycle of increasingly violent confrontations. Ultimately, the process becomes so expensive that all sides lose. The weaker side, unwilling to disengage, may go underground and use terror to frustrate the other side or to get revenge for past injuries. As between the warring peoples of former Yugoslavia or the factions in Northern Ireland, the resolving of such an intense level of conflict becomes very difficult. Referees in national league soccer or basketball games often have to cope with a milder version of this behavior. Thus, two roles that contribute to de-escalating such conflicts are the *buffer-peacekeeper* (to keep the sides apart) and *penalizer* (or activator of sanctions when norms or agreements have been violated).

*Observations.* Personal or collective violence may lead to conflicts that persist for hundreds of years. They are exemplified by the recurring wars of ethnic or tribal groups like those in former Yugoslavia, Sudan, or Rwanda.

## NINE PROFESSIONAL
## CONFLICT RESOLUTION ROLES

Earlier in this chapter, professional conflict resolution roles were seen as definitive. In actual practice, some characteristics of one role (e.g., facilitator) may overlap partly with another (say, of mediator or healer). Furthermore, the interpersonal or situational demands of resolving a conflict may require the intervention of a team of diversely talented professionals (Keasly and Fisher 1990; Ross and Lappin 1967; Rothman 1974). Certain basic skills may be shared by a number of role-players, but even if the intervener is a single person, a number of professional roles seem essential if we are to cope effectively with the five types of conflict mentioned above.

Nine focal roles are elaborated below:

### Facilitator

Essentially, facilitators help the parties in a disagreement to keep communications open among participants as well as between them and important actors in their environment. While staying clear of deep emotional feelings, the facilitator's intent is to remove the obstacles to direct communication between the parties. As in most labor-management negotiations, facilitators help promote existing linkages and relationships by penetrating closed boundaries and by clarifying misunderstandings that have blocked the communication channels. They often re-emphasize to all parties how much all of them have in common, as well as coach them about outcomes that can meet the needs of the other side as well as satisfy their own needs.

In 1992-1993, when both the Israeli government and the PLO leadership came to a similar dissatisfaction with business as usual, they were able to utilize the help of Norwegian facilitators. The latter provided meeting places and took care of all vital technical arrangements during the months of secret talks that led to the signing of a peace agreement. As vital as the facilitation was, its practitioners do not take a direct part either in the negotiations or in policy determination.

### Healer

Conflict resolving may require the involvement of a social therapist or healer. Operating at the community level, the healer investigates the underlying causes of a continuing conflict, and begins an appropriate kind of treatment through group representatives or leaders (Ross and Lappin 1967). This may require looking at taboo ideas, overcoming historical hatreds, verbalizing feelings of deprivation or suffering, departing from traditional beliefs or customs, discontinuing behavior that humiliates or victimizes other groups, improving self-understanding, and listening sensitively to the complaints of the other side.

A healer will know, for example, that if people have been forcibly isolated in ghetto-like enclaves, if they are obsessed with dangers to their own survival, if their children attend substandard inner-city schools, if they have been brutalized in captivity, or if they have been denied opportunities to participate in decisions that impact critically on the conduct of their lives, they are likely to be full of rage. Similarly, if faced by a serious scarcity of vital resources or a threat to their security, vulnerable people can be paralyzed with fear. Persons or organizations characterized by so much fear and anger tend to be righteous and fanatic in their outlook. In negotiation sessions, they are likely to distrust rather than take risks, monopolize rather than share, and manipulate rather than cooperate.

With the help of a trusted third-party healer, both sides can learn a nonjudgmental way of interrelating. An empathic healer will listen to both the content and the affect expressed by participants, focus on their expressions of need, and enable them to hear each other more effectively. Being listened to is a basic preliminary to the development of interpersonal trust and of willingness to reexamine issues (Frank and Ascher 1951; Kelman 1991; Peck 1993). With supportive help, expressions of regret or forgiveness can eventually be communicated clearly, and can bring about enough general catharsis to enable a peace-making process to start or resume (Knudson-Hoffman 1993; Montville 1987 and 1989b; Wallis 1993).

In fact, a healer such as the psychiatrist Carl Rogers brought together military and political leaders in relatively isolated settings (away from the mass media), in order to encounter each other as human beings (Rogers and Ryback 1984). During these types of meetings, they listened actively to each others' grievances and wounds, put strong feelings into words, appreciated the other side's version of historic events, tried to understand normal responses to hurts and losses, and (in such a safe environment) gave expression to contrition and forgiveness. When it is relevant, people can be helped to gain insight into the impact of dehumanizing "the enemy." Ultimately, the catharsis of a full mourning process sets both sides free from the absolutist ideological slogans that usually escalate conflicts toward mutual violence (Montville 1993; Rosenheck 1985).

Healing processes have transformed relationships between Israelis and Egyptians, the Germans and the French (after World War II), Japanese and Americans, etc. They have brought about the cessation of urban gang wars (Wallis 1993). In contrast, when healing processes fail to take place, the outcomes are vicious wars such as those between the Croats and the Serbs, the Kurds and the Turks, government forces and Jonas Savimbi's Unita forces (in the civil war in Angola), the Cambodian government and the Khmer Rouge, Iraq and Iran, the Zulus and their ANC rivals in South Africa, or the Tutsi and the Hutu tribes in Rwanda.

## *Mediator*

The professional mediator often works to enhance a committee process or the functioning of local leaders. This type of intervention teaches the parties how to take notice of the demands of all the interest groups (including those that may not have reached the negotiating table). Mediators try to function objectively, but they are seldom neutral. They have a strong desire to bring about a successful resolution of the conflict and are usually committed to a definite set of professional values (Parsons 1991).

In fact, a mediator functions best in conflict situations where the disputants know each other, desire to engage in ongoing interactions, are still open-minded, and control similar quantities of power or resources. Under such constraints, skilled mediators try to encourage face-to-face contacts, help the rivals focus on specific issues, and encourage a free airing of grievances or differences of interests. The mediator often softens the edge of a controversy by acting as a reliable conduit of information, as a translator-interpreter of difficult messages, or as a censor of the unacceptable (Cohen 1990). Just as the enabler in social work, the conflict mediator strengthens the functioning of all participants, until they are able to use a participatory process to solve their problem.

A few examples of the rich literature of mediation will have to suffice here. Warren (1964) used his experience in mediating between East and West Germany to suggest that the mediator can be an agent for reconciliation in most intersystemic conflicts. Mediation has been used successfully to resolve disagreements between divorcing family members (Weingarten and Douvan 1985), with the parties in child-custody cases (Pearson and Thoennes 1985), in neighborhood tensions (Shonholz 1984), and consumer-merchant disputes (Chandler 1985).

*Expert-Consultant*

In a contest or competitive environment, professionals often function as nonpartisan experts or consultants (Andrews 1991). If local mediation staff have good reasons not to play this role personally, they may well import an outside expert to get the job done. Large business or industrial organizations often use OD (organization development) consultants to help make their operations more efficient.

Generally, as exemplified by Henry Kissinger Associates today, experts do not take part in the process of settling a conflict that may follow their advice giving. Their focus remains on "educating" the participants to a higher level of understanding, in order to set the stage for a reduction of misunderstandings and of partisan quarreling.

For example, in 1992, especially as Israel began to prepare for the Madrid peace talks, a change of policy took place in the Ministry of Education. Some visionaries became aware that Israel might, in the near future, be forced to live with its former Arab enemies as neighbors. After years of defensive wars and being strong militarily, many pupils and some teachers in Israel's school system lacked the attitudes, knowledge, or skills essential for living in peace. In the near future, Israelis of all ages would need to learn how to be at peace with themselves, how to engage in meaningful dialogue with former enemies, and how to understand the complexities of compromising in order to achieve mutually satisfying agreements. Cultivating a sense of optimism seemed desirable. This meant re-examining some of the basic concepts of Judaism, Zionism, and democracy.

In January 1993, I was invited to give consultation to the Unit for Democracy and Coexistence of the Ministry of Education. In order to help Israelis get ready for "an era of peace," I introduced a group of top staff of that Unit to existing materials in the English language, and they decided to translate various full or partial curriculum items into Hebrew.

*Advocate*

When one side in a conflict is so weak or so demoralized that it cannot contend with the stronger party (e.g., an ethnically stigmatized poverty neighborhood that has been neglected or manipulated by City Hall politicians for many years), the situation calls for an advocate. Such a tough-minded professional identifies partisanly with the weaker side and uses a range of tactics to stop the stronger party from continuing to benefit from current inequalities. The advocate will exploit legalities, confront, offer the news media a juicy scoop, try to create or sustain a crisis environment, threaten to go to higher authorities, and sometimes make creative use of public embarrassment on behalf of the victimized groups (Alinsky 1946; Brager 1968; Chetkow 1968; Netting and Hinds 1984).

Parallel to getting the exploiter to pay attention to the victims' demands, advocates usually teach their clients how the system works, how to make choices for themselves, and how to learn skills of assertiveness in negotiating (Schneiderman 1965). After the weak have been strengthened and the overstrong restrained, former victims are expected to be able to take care of themselves. Advocates are skilled risk takers. They often use the establishment's own tactics as a means for achieving immediate justice or for bringing about significant change (see following case example).

*Arbitrator*

Sometimes the conflict environment is so polarized that making progress requires a clearly directive role such as arbitrator. When the parties cannot resolve issues themselves, but do not wish to resort to violence, they search for a mutually acceptable authoritarian person or institution (a retired judge or court process). They tell their stories separately to the person in charge and agree to abide by whatever the arbitrator decides. This is what happened between Egypt and Israel when they could not agree about the disposal of the Taba region along their new border.

## Administrator

After the parties to a conflict have reached an agreement, there is still much to be done, and the role of administrator or implementer becomes vital. Not only must the terms of the agreement be made operational, but each phase or development must be monitored. If difficulties arise, the original intentions of the signatories may require interpretation or redefining. Talented administrators will try to mold public opinion, as well as to stay in touch with opinion makers and political leaders of all sides. They work sensitively to prevent the emergence of new misunderstandings that could lead to a new cycle of escalation.

When appropriate, administrators may be required to create new options for implementing a treaty's provisions, and for renewing educational encounter-meetings between the parties or their descendants (Mitchell 1991) . The implementation phase is successful if what was once a conflict situation is transformed into an altered reality–one in which a new or renewed consensus-cooperation prevails (Warren 1972; Chetkow-Yanoov 1992).

## Buffer

When the interaction is very intense, or it has escalated to such a level of negativity that those involved no longer want to achieve resolution but rather desire to destroy their opponent, an important role to be filled is that of buffer or separator. The buffer does not engage in reconciliatory activities. When there is danger of an exchange of blows between parliament members whose debating has become personal and heated, someone interposes physically between them in order to keep them from doing something they will later regret, or simply to stop them from doing each other harm. Often the short pause created gives each side an opportunity to cool off. The United Nations' peacekeeping force in Sinai filled this kind of function by separating Egyptian and Israeli armed forces.

*Penalizer*

In some traditional societies, norm-violating hotheads, or enemies, are "isolated" by means of excommunication. They may be "cursed" by a professional (as in the Biblical story of Balaam), or have voodoo powers invoked against them.

A contemporary version of punishing norm-violating countries is to mount economic sanctions against them, as the United Nations did in the case of Iraq after it attacked Kuwait. When (white-dominated) South African behaviors became normative again, the sanctions were canceled.

## A CASE EXAMPLE

The case described below, a composite of a number of projects, includes several professional conflict resolution roles. Basically, the episode took place within an old, high-density, racially mixed, lower middle-class neighborhood, on the outer fringe of the inner city of an American metropolitan region. Once a neighborhood of great prestige, tree-lined boulevards, large yards, and contiguous to a university campus, it now showed many signs of abandonment and neglect. City Hall had just closed its last remaining youth center there. The neighborhood had to contend with daily masses of urban traffic streaming from the suburbs to city center in the morning and back every evening. Lately, the area's in-mobility rate had risen sharply, especially with regard to younger African-American families with many children. At night, the streets were jammed with parked cars. All the public schools were overcrowded (Chetkow 1968).

As the coordinator of the area's Neighborhood Association, I received a phone call one morning from Mrs. C, who complained that her block was being torn up by a road construction company. Big chunks of cement were lying all around, mud was everywhere, and huge machines were left unattended at night—posing a real danger to neighborhood children and preventing residents from parking near their homes. No attempt had been made to give the neighbors notice that the project was to begin, nor to discuss compensation for shrubs, grass, and trees removed by bulldozers. Work crew members were close-mouthed, and behaved very rudely toward neighbors who asked them what was going on.

My contacts within the Planning Department confirmed that Metropolis was extending a one-way traffic pattern throughout the southern tip of the neighborhood. During the afternoon, I phoned one of my friends in the mayor's office, who was already informed about the situation. As a member of the same political party, I stressed that we were going to lose a lot of votes, and that the neighbors were already talking about going to the mass media. She asked me to stay cool, and promised to talk both to the city engineer and the mayor. I said that I could not be "cool" if some child fell into a mud hole or broke an arm on the cement chunks that were lying around.

Two days later, nothing had changed. The city engineer was so evasive that I told him I intended to "go over his head." I called my friend in the mayor's office, and letting the anger in my voice be heard clearly, asked her to do something before the Association calls the newspapers or helps the neighbors to sue the city. . . . In the meantime, Mrs. C called to report that many of her neighbors were very upset. I suggested that she call some of them together for a meeting. I would be ready to help them write a letter of complaint, and to get the Neighborhood Association to write one as well.

When I arrived at Mrs. C's house after supper, a noisy group of residents were hard at work. They were united in their bitterness against City Hall—both about the messed-up streets and the closing of their youth center (while their teens were dropping out of school and on the verge of delinquency). Enough of the neighbors had grown up together in this integrated area, and were now active in the same political party, so that they were ready to do something. I led an intensive group discussion for over two hours, helping people express their outrage as well as building a bridge between those who wanted to go to court and others who suggested that we try meeting with city representatives first. After listening to each other, they agreed to undertake a number of protest steps, and that they wanted to do this as a subcommittee of the Neighborhood Association.

The next few days were very busy. They accepted my offer to help them design and conduct a quick survey of their neighbors' opinions and desires. I suggested ways they might make a visit to the city engineer, and offered to get them a session with the mayor. Some of them were ready to start up a parent-run youth center in Mrs. C's basement. They were pleased to learn that a grant might be obtained for this purpose from a local charitable foundation, and the process was begun.

Through my friend in the mayor's office, immediate meetings were scheduled for our protesters to meet with the city engineer and the mayor himself. On the day of those meetings, the neighbors (whom I had rehearsed the day before) handled these encounters by themselves. They were very firm with the engineer, so that he made some concessions and promised to talk to the bosses of the road-building company. The mayor was surprised at how much these citizen voters knew about city business and at the polite firmness they displayed. He agreed to have the city's Human Rights Commission set up, and mediate, a series of meetings with representatives of the Neighborhood Association, starting the following week.

When the mayor heard that these citizens were already seeking funding advice in order to organize their own youth center, he called his budget director and instructed her to look into the possibility of reactivating the neighborhood's youth center.

Within the next three weeks, four meetings with the Neighborhood Association did take place, mediated skillfully by the director of the Human Rights Commission. Three weeks later, the roads were rehabilitated and paved, street lights restored, and sidewalks added. The construction crews were reported to be polite, showing concern for children's safety. When the reactivation of the youth center became a distinct possibility, leaders were recruited to organize a Scout Troop, and after-school tutoring sessions were scheduled.

## IMPLICATIONS

Even though most conflict-resolving roles imply a process of de-escalating the interaction from actual or potential violence toward compromise or consensus, not every human-relations professional is able to perform all these roles. Twenty years ago, organizational analysis suggested that work settings influence the role expectations of social-worker change agents toward employing or avoiding conflict resolution strategies. Professionals who are agency oriented usually favor status quo norms and avoid conflict. In contrast, an orientation toward clients can have a radicalizing impact on professional functioning. Workers with this orientation are comfortable using confrontation strategies. Interestingly, being oriented strictly to the profession is neither conservatizing nor radicalizing (Epstein 1970).

For organizations or practitioners who take conflict resolution seriously, intervention roles also vary in accordance with such considerations as:

1. the stage of escalation (from consensus to violence) to which the conflict has evolved;
2. whether the intervention is geared to settling a substantive issue (e.g., who is to control a specific territory), to improving relationships (e.g., between the Protestants and Catholics of Northern Ireland), or both;
3. whether or not helper roles are structured in a series (e.g., varying from nondirective facilitation to highly directive arbitration). In addition, successful resolution of conflicts may well require the simultaneous employment of a multitalented team of intervenors—so that a wide range of skills are available simultaneously; and
4. whether the intervention efforts are geared to reducing ignorance, or to easing the fear and rage that accompany repeated victimization and deprivation.

Generally, substantive issues can be managed by reducing ignorance and focusing on logical procedures. Easing powerful emotions requires a very different set of skills (see above discussion of the healer role).

We suggest another way to analyze the range of professional roles required for resolving a community conflict productively.

In a serious but nonviolent clash, vulnerable or weak participants may require the immediate services of a *buffer* and/or an *advocate*.

Both sides are likely to respond to the suggestions of an empathetic *healer*. Once that phase has been accomplished, a skilled *facilitator*, armed with *expert* advice, can help the groups get their act together, set action goals, and look for resources to make action possible. During the regular process of disagreement, it is common to seek the help of a *mediator*. In really difficult situations (e.g., of power imbalance and/or fanaticism), both sides may agree to accept help from an *arbitrator*. Once the conflict has been resolved and the desired outcomes agreed to, the services of a skilled *administrator* become useful.

During conflicts in which neither norms nor interim agreements have been violated, the services of a *penalizer* are not likely to be required.

## SUMMARY

This chapter focused on nine kinds of professional roles and how they might be appropriate for various kinds of conflict situations. Of course, each type or level of conflict requires interventions appropriate to its dynamics. The sophisticated choreographing of appropriate professional roles and interventions can reverse escalation—preventing a conflict from becoming violent or destructive. Fortunately, the art and science of conflict resolution have matured in the past 20 years. Today, many of the skills required to do the above can be learned, and have shown themselves to be effective.

In the following chapter, we shall try to understand how the work of the professional conflict resolver might be supplemented by volunteers.

Chapter 8

# The Role of Volunteers
# in Conflict Resolution

## *INTRODUCTION*

In the pre-state years of many countries, most social services were provided by volunteers. Since formal social services and the helping professions did not exist during such periods, most mutual aid originated from the family, groups of neighbors, religious institutions, or public-spirited benefactors. Remnants of this early tradition are still exemplified in volunteer-operated fire departments, Red Cross services, Alcoholics Anonymous, or the Salvation Army. Before the professionalization of social work, home visits for counseling, leisure opportunities, and social reform were performed by socially concerned citizens.

For social workers, the issue of a public/voluntary division of labor began with Mary Richmond. Back in 1913, as public services and the helping professions were in their infancy, she warned the social workers of her day to be ready for a period of readjustment, and in 1930 she found it necessary to make a strong case for the continuing importance of volunteers (Richmond 1971). In fact, with the passage of time, voluntarism shifted from something sporadic and unorganized to a continuous kind of systematized activity. Formal tasks, defined as appropriate to the volunteer, were distinguished from those of the qualified professional.

Voluntary agencies also became an integral part of the human-service landscape. Today volunteers contribute significantly in such fields as health, youth, corrections, leisure, immigrant absorption, education, civil defense, social planning, and environmental protection. The simple voluntary agencies of the early part of the century have evolved into influential semi-establishment nongovernmental organizations (NGOs), and flourish amid the efforts of larger public services.

In recent years, scholars have refined the differences between services offered by governmental or public, market-oriented or for-profit, religious or philanthropic, and self-help auspices. Moreover, some public agencies merely pay lip service to the idea of using volunteers. Having come full circle, contemporary service professionals are often hostile toward volunteers, and actually seem to be threatened by their presence (Gidron 1983). It is still unclear whether voluntary services should relate to the public services as competitors, should supplement them, or whether they should complement one another.

## PUBLIC/VOLUNTARY RESPONSIBILITY FOR CONFLICT RESOLUTION

Much has been written on the ideal public/voluntary division of labor in urban-industrial Western society. Three major service-auspices are commonly mentioned:

| GOVERNMENTAL DEPARTMENTS | VOLUNTEER ACTIVITIES | PROFIT-MAKING OPERATIONS |
|---|---|---|
| Guaranteed rights in a welfare state | Criticize, advocate, innovate | Sell what has proved popular |
| Control | Independence | Making profits |
| Standards/norms | Pluralism | Free market |
| Tax funds | Donations | User fees |
| Universal coverage | For special or weak populations | For those who pay the costs |
| Monitoring, and implementing whatever the law authorizes | Flexibility and pioneering amidst fragmentation, accountability | Deregulation, function very efficiently, copy others |

Scholars (e.g., Kramer 1985) argue that many of the above governmental/voluntary, voluntary/commercial, or governmental/commercial dichotomies are not valid today. In postindustrial Western societies, both voluntary and public services have become elitistic and bureaucratized, and both primarily protect their "turfs." Consequently, we have seen a rapid development of grassroots or participatory networks, cooperatives, and self-help groups. Local citizens now participate in neighborhood renewal projects, boards of cooperative nursery schools, high schools, neighborhood associations, food-purchasing cooperatives, councils, and coalitions.

Today, both public and voluntary service agencies are seen as legally limited in what they have to offer, even uncaring. Unwilling to remain dependent upon a centralized establishment, people in neighborhoods expect authority to flow upward from the grass roots (as in self-help groups and social networks) rather than downward from centralistic power structures.

## VOLUNTARY ARAB-JEWISH RECONCILIATION

In order to look at the functioning of a voluntary organization in this delicate area, a short review of some recent Israeli history is helpful.

### A Minihistory of Recent Arab-Jewish Tensions within Israel

Some 100 years of hostility have made a deep impact on both Israel's Jewish and Arab populations. Because many of Israel's Jewish citizens have survived either the Holocaust in Europe or other persecutions in Arab countries-of-origin, they feel and act like victims (in line with the model outlined in Chapter 5). Attacks by armies of surrounding Arab countries, as well as acts of violence/terror perpetrated within the borders of Israel, reawaken the trauma of past Nazi, Moslem, Christian, and other historic persecutions. Jewish immigrants to Israel, and later their children, became engaged in a repetitive pattern of wars, border clashes, terrorist infiltrations, hijackings, etc. Vast amounts of scarce economic resources were diverted from construction and social service purposes in order to maintain a defense establishment.

Few Jews noticed how urbanization and modernization were changing the predominantly village lifestyle of the Arab population of Israel. Even though the public schools (and other social services) of the country's Palestinian citizens were segregated and inferior to those of Jewish citizens, a generation of Israel-educated young

Arabs came into adulthood. This new intelligentsia began to challenge traditional village leadership, to evolve a positive self-identity and a national commitment, and to relate to their fellow (Jewish) citizens as equals.*

They began to demand their rights as citizens, but many Jewish politicians and/or bureaucrats continued to treat them as second-class citizens. This, along with anti-Arab violence by Jewish fanatics and unfulfilled promises of help from Arab countries in the Middle East, created a parallel sense of victimization on the part of Israel's Arab population. In such a charged environment, any small incident would send both sides into crisis, or stir up a backlash of angry violence.

During these same years, while normal channels for Arab-Jewish contact lessened, enlightened persons on both sides realized the importance of working out a pragmatic form of coexistence. Courageous Jewish and Arab members of Israel's nonestablishment peace movement became more active during the past twenty years, and continue now–despite the Intifada, the "war" in the Persian Gulf, and subsequent acts of terror by suicidal chamas Moslems (in bus bombings, etc.) and fanatic Jews such as Dr. Goldstein (who shot Moslems at prayer in Hebron).

As the peace movement became more sophisticated, it began using such strategies as:

1. redefining the (Arab-Jewish) problem or condition;
2. engaging in advocacy on behalf of current victims;
3. recruiting new activists within the Jewish establishment;
4. creating voluntary organizations for grassroots dialogue;
5. scheduling protest rallies and confrontations;
6. financing demonstration projects of reconciliation; and
7. designing ways to teach peacemaking skills in schools.

Slowly, skilled staff persons began to function on the edge of politics, attempting small projects of social action or conflict resolution (Chetkow-Yanoov 1988).

---

*The dual national identity of Israel's Palestinian citizens, especially since the outbreak of the Intifada in 1987, is too complex a topic to be dealt with here.

## ONE VOLUNTARY WAY:
## THE "PARTNERSHIP" ASSOCIATION

As part of the above peace movement, I functioned as an activist-citizen and leader within a small voluntary organization of Arabs and Jews based primarily in the Haifa area. As an organization, it was independent of all branches of government and for many years also politically nonpartisan. Supported by interested persons and groups in Israel and from other countries, its entire budget came from philanthropic contributors and foundations in Israel and abroad.

This organization was created by a number of professional educators and a Baptist pastor in 1975. Both the Jewish and Arab founders, having grown tired of demonstrations and protests, came to the conclusion that efforts should be invested in moving from relationships of unwilling dependency on "an enemy" into one of interdependence or partnership with a new friend (formerly seen as the enemy). Experts in their own fields, the founders decided to devote the organization's few resources to making a master plan for resettling the residents of an Arab village dislocated by the country's War of Independence. They also pioneered the first formal peace curriculum (for Israel's Jewish high schools), developed a model for training leaders for mixed experiential groups, and tried to create a mechanism for coordinating their work with that of other peace organizations (Chetkow-Yanoov 1986).

The organization was formally incorporated in 1977. Its incorporation papers insisted on Arab and Jewish co-chairpersons, a mixed board of directors, as well as Jewish and Arab employees. Gradually a transition took place, from a group of concerned experts to a small-scale social movement. This led to a shift from relating to objective problems toward a focus on interpersonal and psychological ones.

Between 1977 and 1979, members came to realize that work on human feelings (such as helplessness, anger, or fear) was needed, and it became part of training sessions that allowed mutual support by colleagues. Many intensive human-relations group processes, especially in the format of weekend workshops, were scheduled–in order to overcome our own prejudices, learn to trust the motives of the other side, experience aspects of each other's cultures, and develop skills for engaging in broad educational projects promoting coexistence.

After 1979, the organization underwent still another transition, from a volunteer movement to a formally registered nonprofit association. It then functioned with the help of trained activist members and a small professional staff. By then, its constitution included the following goal statements:

1. to enhance conditions of communications and partnership between Israeli Jews and Arabs;
2. to do everything possible to prevent situations that might give rise to conflicts of interest or to mutual distrust among Jews and Arabs; and
3. to coordinate activities with individuals and other organizations working toward similar goals.

Over the subsequent years of trial and error, Association leaders and activists learned that one of the most effective ways to convert former enemies into partners involved creating new ways to work together in an atmosphere of growing mutual trust. Efforts were devoted to learning intergroup skills, and to spreading the approach to others through conference papers, workshops, simulations, and weekend seminars. Under field conditions, contacts were fostered through interschool class-to-class minipartnerships, three-day intercommunity workshops, adult discussion evenings, and mixed summer camps.

By 1982, Association board members realized that educational activities must be supplemented by efforts to bring about community change. Independent of local or national public services, it started a social development project in a lower-class neighborhood of Haifa marked by a complete absence of communication between its Jewish and Arab residents. Because many of the Jewish residents were elderly Holocaust survivors, they were afraid of Arabs, and earlier Arab initiatives had ended in failure. Claiming lack of budget, City Hall had just closed down a youth center, the only existing social service in the Arab part of the neighborhood. Educational facilities for the Arab children were also of low standard.

Some of the Association's younger Arab members, who lived in the area, brought the situation to the board's attention. Eventually, the Association decided to work in this neighborhood. A professional social worker was employed to explore the situation. She soon discovered that the Arab residents, although angry and fearful about the future of their children, were open to contact with Jews. She began a series of weekly meetings with concerned Arab residents—which developed into a quasitherapeutic relationship for several months. Toward the end of this period, the Arab residents felt secure enough to form a neighborhood association.

During the following year, they began to plant gardens around their buildings, They were helped to raise some funds, became an official nonprofit organization, opened their own youth center, and started a kindergarten for the children of the area's working mothers. At this point, the City was embarrassed into reinstating the Arab youth center, and negotiations took place (with the worker's quiet guidance) to ensure that the residents retained control of their own new agencies. Once the Arab residents began to feel more confident, beginning contacts were made with the Jewish residents about neighborhood problems that were common to both Jews and Arabs.

The Association also helped set up a comprehensive intervention project in a mixed neighborhood of Acre. This project involved a combination of community action and education, meetings with city and national bureaucrats, supplying expert consultants, finding and training grassroots leaders, holding work camps, making contacts with news media, and helping fledgling citizen associations to obtain funds in order to expand the scope of their activities.*

## OTHER VOLUNTARY
## CONFLICT RESOLUTION EFFORTS

Parallel to the evolution of voluntary social services, sophisticated citizens are learning how to handle local conflicts without the assistance of governmental agencies (Edelson 1981). In an impoverished neighborhood of San Francisco, for example, residents were trained to function as volunteer arbitrators and mediators of grassroots conflicts (Shonholz 1984). Participants, recruited directly from the neighborhood, undergo two weeks of training (usually

---

*It should be noted that after the Intifada began, the Association became overly identified with Israel's political left. This change of focus caused it to lose its access to the public school system.

managed by other volunteers). They emerge able to conduct out-reach, manage cases, serve as panelists, and accomplish follow-up. Not only has this Neighborhood Justice System become a valuable alternative to the criminal justice system, it helps resolve interneighbor conflicts, and also provides local activists with opportunities for personal growth and skills learning. This approach has proved viable in urban, suburban, rural, and tribal settings (Brager and Jarin 1969; Mansfield 1988; Rogers 1990).

### Seniors Help Mediate Local Conflicts

Most of us are aware that for many elders, retirement poses problems of excessive free time, and in serious cases, dangers of social disengagement caused by loss of former social roles. Since many retirees have accumulated valuable knowledge and occupational skills, the challenge is to create new roles for them. Today, unsophisticated elders can be seen functioning as crossing guards at busy intersections, as grandfatherly assistants in nursery schools, or as living repositories of modern history. Former judges, professors, business executives, social workers, etc., are finding satisfaction in offering their services in voluntary-agency settings and in antipoverty programs.

One of the exciting new roles evolving for healthy retirees is conflict mediators—especially for elders who get into trouble with unethical commercial establishments, with neighbors in large apartment buildings, or with ageism and prejudice. Cox and Parsons (1992) report a model project started in Denver (United States). Retired persons (average age 72) volunteered for this project, underwent rigorous training, and worked in teams of two for a period of nine months. They were able to mediate conflicts that elders had with neighbors, concerning tenants' rights, with unsavory business operators, with legal issues, and with sexual abuse.

Both the "clients" they helped and the volunteer "practitioners" themselves reported high levels of satisfaction. The latter found they could project trust well enough to help contending elders to work out a satisfactory agreement. They also found they could apply their new skills to their own lives.

## *Multitrack Diplomacy for Resolving Conflicts*

Along with the growing awareness that peace for one nation is interdependent with the fate of other nations, conflict resolution practitioners have begun to recognize the idea of multitrack diplomacy (Diamond and McDonald 1991). Although international diplomacy is conducted directly by officials and diplomats of sovereign governments and by United Nations staff, a variety of conflict resolution activities also take place outside such formal channels. Individual professional, academic, business, mass media, religious and nongovernmental-funding bodies are increasingly involved in unofficial-informal activities to reduce or resolve world-level conflicts.

One example of volunteer diplomacy is that of the American Friends Service Committee's efforts to reduce conflicts in many parts of the world. Since it was founded in 1917, the AFSC

> has carried out extensive relief and social service work–especially for refugees of the many armed conflicts that have marked this century. In the last 25 to 30 years, the AFSC has been trying to establish the conditions of peace through informal, off-the-record diplomatic conferences, student exchanges and missions to trouble spots in times of tension. Because of the backlog of good will created by its service activities, the AFSC has been quite successful in its quiet diplomacy. . . . The AFSC, as a general procedure, keeps the [U.S.] State Department informed about [its] activities. However, AFSC officials, to establish their credibility as mediators, must be clearly perceived as independent private citizens and completely neutral. (Warren 1987)

Another example comes out of the peace movement in Israel. A number of NGOs working in the field of peace education were able to create attractive curriculum materials that were accepted as elective teaching materials by the Ministry of Education. Not only did these volunteer operations turn Arab-Jewish encounter meetings into educational experiences, but ways were brainstormed to accomplish similar outcomes by means of computer contacts between schools. When the Ministry, in the post-Madrid era of peace talks, wanted to prepare the entire Israeli school system for an era of peace, staff from its Unit on Democracy and Coexistence sought consultation from faculty members of various universities.

A third multitrack example was, in fact, the year-long process that led to the recent peace treaty between the Israeli government and the PLO. In summer of 1992, a Norwegian trade union team came to Israel in order to research Palestinian living conditions. The team was headed by a sociologist who developed trust relationships with Israeli governmental and PLO officials. It became clear that both sides wanted to set up a secret channel for direct Israel-PLO talks. One member of the research team happened to be the wife of Norway's foreign minister.

With such academic and political connections, secret meetings were soon taking place in Norway and other places in Europe. The official peace talks (which had started in Madrid in October 1991 and subsequently moved to Washington, DC) were stalled, but this secret channel produced the breakthrough formula of "Gaza and Jericho first" in eleven months. Of course, prime minister Rabin and foreign minister Peres were involved, and took an active part in using this unofficial Norwegian channel as well as a formal Egyptian one (Susser 1992).

## SOME ADVANTAGES
## OF USING VOLUNTARY AUSPICES

In a highly politicized society such as Israel, both Jewish and Arab members of the previously described Association found a way to do something without becoming another political party. Their voluntary auspices provided them an effective way for expressing discontent and for investing energy in corrective counter-measures. Being active in such a "safe" setting made possible the reduction of fear or anger and the working out of feelings of guilt.

Private individuals and NGOs–functioning as facilitators, mediators, and expert consultants–are able to lower tension by means of direct encounters across ethnic or national boundaries. After they develop trust and credibility with their informal counterparts, they utilize their considerable skills and expertise to explore new ways for dealing with troublesome regional conflicts. Of course, as private persons, they can take risks (i.e., cross "taboo" borders) as well as function without the need to display special reverence for the official policies of their governments. With adequate private resources, they can persist over long periods of time. Within networks of mutual support, they have been known to exert significant influence on the policies or actions of their own governments (Boulding 1990; McDonald and Bendahmane 1987).

Voluntary peace organizations provide legitimate work-settings for talented Arab as well as Jewish young persons. The Association hired a number of its former program participants, and some of them eventually became members of its Board of Directors. Former Arab as well as Jewish activists have used the skills and insights that they accumulated during Association activities in successful careers as physicians, educators, administrators, and clergy.

Kramer (1981) is but one of many scholars who strongly advocate that social change be achieved through voluntary auspices. Thus, in the realities of Arab-Jewish relations in Israel, legal and financial independence from both local governments and from all political party establishments enable voluntary associations to innovate new services and approaches. Sophisticated and well-motivated citizens have negotiated delicate issues with branches of the establishment, as Association board members did with the Ministry of Education. When government officials as well as volunteers are seen as partners rather than enemies, informal cooperative relations become the basis for effective experimentation and pioneering.

Two concrete examples of success in this field occurred during the past decade in Israel. A voluntary organization of parents with mentally disabled children lobbied successfully to expand the law's coverage–so that the term "handicapped" included mental as well as physical disability. The Haifa Association's master plan for returning Arab refugees to their evacuated village on Israel's northern border was another social action or lobbying effort by a voluntary auspice on behalf of a distressed population group. The effort had reached as far as a meeting between the Association team and the Minister of the Treasury, when elections caused the existing Labor government to be replaced by the Likud party, and the project died.

When working with high officials of public establishments, the voluntary organization must have something valuable to offer in exchange for cooperation or support. The offer of pedagogic or human relations expertise for teachers' training, of seed money for small demonstration projects, or of a well-prepared activity often proves attractive to responsible bureaucrats. Devoting resources to necessary tiresome homework in order to be able to suggest a better plan for accomplishing a specific goal (rather than merely blaming or criticizing) often generates a positive response. In fact, when a citizen lobby does achieve legislative change (due to its contribution of volunteer time, energy, and knowledge), this is often a result of quiet cooperation from those who administer the relevant governmental service (Addams 1983; Andrews 1991; Schottland 1966).

Voluntary associations are able to go beyond the requirements of the law, i.e., to undertake projects which the law does not prohibit. For example, long-range Arab-Jewish reconciliation by means of public school studies is desirable, but not enough. Formal classroom lessons in tolerance and coexistence should be supplemented with voluntary efforts to teach parallel messages to parents and to other relatives in order to generate a family environment which supports the school's formal efforts. Also, a vanguard or change-agent role can be geared to producing change at the policy level when responsible citizens give testimony or act as a lobby on behalf of a new law. Voluntary organizations should give visible support to controversial programs such as coexistence education in order to counterbalance its opponents who are always vocal in their opposition.

If we wish to live in a world where ideological differences, ethnic rivalries, and/or economic competitions are settled by means of negotiation and bargaining rather than by force, we must insist that public and voluntary efforts are themselves based on a true partnership.

## SUMMARY

Voluntary efforts, whether originating at grassroots or elitist levels of the local community, have much to contribute to conflict resolution. Not only can volunteers support the formal thrusts of government agencies, but they often serve as pioneers who explore new areas of conflict resolution. As supplementation for official workers, local activist volunteers appear to be able to advance conflict resolution in many ways.

# PART IV:
# IMPLICATIONS

Chapter 9

# Conflict Resolution Skills
# Can Be Taught

## INTRODUCTION

After I became an Israeli citizen, I experienced a growing urgency to put my social science and social work knowledge into a framework suitable for use with school children. Since it takes a long time to achieve personal maturity, or to learn the skills of intergroup cooperation, I wanted to start teaching conflict resolution in a systematic way as early in the life cycle as possible (Chetkow-Yanoov 1991a).

Furthermore, most human attitudes and behaviors seem to be learned. For example, in my years as a summer camp director, I found that children's fear of water (in the swimming program) was always learned from one of their parents–actually, babies can learn to swim before they can walk. Children learn to be wary of snakes around the age of two. Disrespect for unusual skin color, shape of eyes, or differing religious practices comes later. In the catchy words of the musical *South Pacific:*

> You've got to be taught to be afraid
> of people whose eyes are oddly made
> and people whose skin is a different shade
> you've got to be carefully taught.

Similarly, years of formal and informal socialization teach us to respond aggressively to real or imagined attacks, and to use violence or go to war when faced with demands or threats.

These various considerations motivated me to participate in the development of four different curricula for teaching conflict resolution in the Israeli public schools.

## THE CONTRIBUTION OF EDUCATION
## TO CONFLICT RESOLUTION

Contemporary social science contends that human nature is not intrinsically violent or warlike (Avruch and Black 1990; Clark 1990). If we must be taught to be wary of strangers, or to be anti-Semitic, racist, sexist, or ageist, we can also be socialized to trust, to appreciate others unlike ourselves, to cooperate, and to respect the law. We can learn how to negotiate, to mediate, to compromise, to share, and to bargain in conflict situations.

Since the public schools have long helped socialize young persons into roles and attitudes considered essential for adult citizenship, formal education efforts must now prepare young persons, adults, and seniors for a peaceful lifestyle within a framework of pluralism. For this, the incremental processes of education are central (I. Harris 1988). It is also important that peace education be initiated in stable settings such as a university, and that such efforts receive a level of prestige commensurate with that of our national military academies.

At the fourth conference of the World Council for Curriculum and Instruction (which took place in Edmonton, Canada in 1984), a keynote speech suggested that while education attempts to be non-partisan, it cannot stay neutral between justice and injustice, cooperation and domination, or between peace and violence. Education that does not emphasize the importance of intergroup understanding and peace is mere training and instruction. In education we must choose whether to socialize into the existing order, or to teach that every social order can be changed. If teachers and pupils learn to conquer situations of fear, oppression, and negative forms of dependence, we may cooperate actively with other people who act the same way–regardless of sex, nation, race, or culture.

## CURRICULUM GOALS

Peace education enterprises call for content and techniques that contribute to the learners' cognitive enrichment, to their practical skills, and to their attitude formation.

Specific learning goals might include:

1. increasing the learners' objective knowledge about the actual diversity of people, viewpoints, and ideologies in their own country, and of the tensions between them;
2. helping learners understand the influence of attitudes and feelings on human behavior in situations of enmity and of cooperation;
3. equipping the learners to analyze the concept "peace" as both a state-of-being and an active process—as well as to enquire into the major obstacles to peacemaking;
4. showing the learners how power can be used to make conflicts escalate (in a variety of family, intergroup, organizational, and community settings), as well as how utilizing nonviolent ways can de-escalate as well as resolve conflicts;
5. helping learners take part in simulations and other participatory learning situations, in order to master some skills and techniques in conflict resolution; and
6. bringing about constructive encounter meetings (and other forms of communication) between members of opposing political parties, religions, ethnic/racial/language groups, social movements—in order to challenge stereotypes, develop trust relationships, develop self-awareness, and search for projects of mutual benefit.

## EIGHT EXAMPLES OF AVAILABLE TEACHING TECHNOLOGIES

So many diverse curricula exist today that it may be difficult to choose among them. For the purposes of this chapter, samples of available teaching materials have been selected on the basis of the age level of their intended learners—from nursery children to older adults. A summary of the basic characteristics of these materials is presented at the conclusion of the chapter.

### Resolving Conflicts in Nursery School

In February 1991, during one of my workshops in South Africa, a local (white) teacher told about a kind of conflict resolution that she initiated in her nursery school. At the beginning of each school year, she introduces her little ones to a special corner that contains an "ear chair," a "mouth chair," and a "friend chair."

When any two children get into a fight, they sit alternatively in the mouth and ear chairs for two minutes. During this time, the mouth person tells his/her side of the problem and the ear person listens silently. After two minutes, they switch chairs, and the former talker now listens to the former listener. If matters have been sufficiently clarified by this process, the two children shake hands and go back to their former activities. If they still feel tense or unhappy, they may invite any other third person (e.g., another pupil, the teacher, the janitor, a parent) to fill the friend chair, and they all talk together until they resolve the conflict.

Our informant explained that this system is generally effective at its basic level, seldom requiring the help of a third person (in the friend chair) to settle the dispute. She was pleased to tell us how comfortably nursery school children internalize the idea that listening to each other works better than hitting or screaming. Although she had not checked personally, she was convinced that the format could be equally effective in black, or integrated nursery schools.

### Languages as a Vehicle to Peacemaking

Concerned citizens in every country might lobby for a national policy that all children be taught two or three languages—their own (local) one and two others. In Israel, for example, all pupils learn Hebrew, Arabic has become compulsory in all the Hebrew-speaking Jewish schools, and all pupils must learn English as a third language. A norm of trilinguality is also found in countries such as Holland or Switzerland. Such a practice, worldwide, would give all children access to another worldview, as well as help them internalize the reality that their group, unique as it is, is not the only one on the planet.

Two scholars have taken the idea one step further. The teaching of the English language can go beyond merely acquiring linguistic skills and communication competence. The curriculum might also guide pupils toward living peacefully with speakers of other languages. Documents, class activities, exercises, etc. can be used to link learning any foreign language with peace education.

In this connection, concerned citizens might insist that all school children be exposed, from the pre-nursery level, to objective information about, as well as to the language of, other ethnic groups living in their region. These groups of language learners should also encounter each other in structured educational situations throughout the grade school and high school years. Parallel sophisticated programs should be set up for their parents—who often have to cope with the ignorance, anger, and fear they have accumulated over a lifetime (Dershowitz 1994; Renner 1994).

We must ensure that existing texts and films—in all programs and curricula—have been cleansed of bigoted stereotypes. Of course, sensitive training programs (often funded by voluntary contributions from abroad) must be arranged each year for classroom personnel who are to teach such innovative curriculum content (Crane 1986, Freudenstein 1992).

### *Fourth Grade Pupils Learn Peer Mediation*

Based on developments in San Francisco (described in Theory Course, Section 6), a team on Canada's west coast developed a set of lessons for fourth grade pupils (Davis 1983; Kalmakoff et al. 1986). This curriculum was the joint product of the teaching staff of a grade school in Burnaby, B.C., of the Public Education for Peace Society of New Westminster, B.C., and of the Faculty of Education of Simon Fraser University, also of Burnaby. Geared to children aged ten, this curriculum includes such content areas as:

Lesson One: CONFLICT

> Definition of conflict.
> Examples of personal conflict situations.
> Analysis of causes of personal conflict.

Lesson Two: CONFLICT RESOLUTION

> Analysis of personal conflict.
> Alternative resolutions to personal conflict situations.
> Win/win resolutions.

Lesson Three: HANDLING ANGER

> Definitions of anger.
> Examples of anger-producing situations.
> Usual angry responses.
> Hurtful and nonhurtful responses.

Lesson Six: IMAGES OF THE ENEMY

> Analysis of hate: How it affects behavior.
> Video: *Neighbors.*
> Transition from conflict on the personal level to conflict on the international level.
> Analysis of causes of international conflict.

Lesson Thirteen: "I CAN DO. . . ."

> Identification of concrete actions for peace.
> Prioritizing actions.
> Cooperative planning of steps toward taking action.

In a stimulating article on "Peaceful Playgrounds," Cheatham (1988) reviewed various efforts to engage school children in mediating classroom and playground disputes. One charming picture shows a grade school girl, wearing a "Conflict Manager" T-shirt, listening intently while mediating between two of her angry male peers. Cheatham approves Tom Roderick's assertion (1987-1988) that resolution of conflicts should become the fourth "R" (along with reading, 'riting, and 'rithmetic) in the curricula of grade and high schools all over the United States. Children who have learned this kind of grassroots peacemaking are expected, later in life, to be able to make connections between their personal conflict management experiences and peacemaking requirements on national and global levels (Brager and Jarin 1969; Fisher and Ury 1983).

### Computerizing the Junior High School Curriculum "Neighbors"

A voluntary association of Jewish and Arab teachers, psychologists, and social workers devoted eight years to producing educational materials on coexistence for Israel's Jewish and Arab junior high schools. Some of the organization's accomplishments include:

1. developing a curriculum of lessons, both in Hebrew and Arabic, for teaching coexistence (knowledge, attitudes, and skills) in Israel's junior high schools. Both the Arabic and the Hebrew texts have been officially approved as a program of choice by the Ministry of Education;
2. holding intensive teacher-training workshops each summer, along with some follow-up workshops during the school year; and
3. pioneering parallel local community workshops for parents of the children in the program.

Between 1984 and 1990, an average of 10,000 Jewish and Arab junior high pupils have studied the curriculum each year.

Although the organization has worked for years to create and improve its "Neighbors" curriculum, the idea of teaching parts of it by means of computers is recent. Social science researchers have demonstrated that if the computer is employed creatively in educational settings, it can serve as a powerful tool for widening students' cognitive processes as well as for improving interpersonal relationships (Fisk and Taylor 1984; Hamilton 1981). Interaction with the computer and with classmates can stimulate such collaborative activities as constructive controversy or sharing of resources. Because learning in such an environment is interactive but at the same time independent of time and distance, it offers educational opportunities which are different from the typical face-to-face classroom.

"Neighbors" started using computers in order to enhance both the cognitive development and intergroup (or intercultural) perceptions of pupils in one Jewish and one Arab junior high school within Israel. A joint team of teachers, "Neighbors" staff, and computer experts met during the summer of 1990, and worked out a basic action-plan for the two schools. During the 1990-1991 school year, volunteer experts prepared a computerized learning-curriculum based on the "Neighbors" program, trained some teachers to use it, and launched it. It was still operating during the 1993-1994 school year.

### *A High School Curriculum: "The Pursuit of Peace"*

On the assumption that distrust, prejudice, and racism are learned behaviors, I prepared a series of lessons to enable the teaching of trust, tolerance, and peaceful ways to resolve conflicts (Chetkow-Yanoov 1985). The principles and skill exercises in each chapter of this book were derived from social work practice as well as from my personal experience in the field of Arab-Jewish reconciliation in Israel during the early 1980s. Many of these lessons later proved relevant in other pluralistic sociocultural settings characterized by intergroup conflict.

The text contains the following chapters:

- Various ways to introduce the topic in a classroom.
- Simulation of the cost of competition vs. cooperation.
- Typical dilemmas in majority-minority relations.
- Defining the concept "peace."
- Hostility, stereotypes, and trust in human relations.
- Victims, victimizers, and archetype behaviors.
- Know your neighbor who lives in the land.
- Games and other cooperative classroom activities.
- What is human nature like?
- Conflict and conflict management.
- How are peace treaties made?
- What the ordinary citizen can do to enhance peace.
- A redefinition of "active" citizenship.
- Findings from the field: Peace studies in practice.
- Going beyond education.

I am convinced that this sort of curriculum, taught by properly trained personnel and backed by school administrators, could equip teenagers with facts, attitudes, and beginning skills for making coexistence work.

Parts and combinations of the above curriculum were tried in the school systems of four Jewish and two Arab municipalities. Some of the basic ideas soon appeared in other educational efforts in Israel, and in a week-long workshop for immigration workers in Sweden. Gradually, I became convinced that the field of peace education can be enhanced by what the social sciences and the helping professions know about human motivation and behavior (Rogers 1965, Burton and Sandole 1986).

### Adults Settle Disputes at the Grassroots Level

As mentioned in the chapter on voluntarism, San Francisco is credited with the *first* training of local residents to function as volunteer mediators of grassroots-level conflicts (Shonholz 1984). This program developed a formal curriculum for training local volunteers to function in conflict resolution panels. A 1984 manual lists such curriculum units as communication skills, outreach, case development, getting cases to hearings, managing the panel during hearings, and advanced conflict resolution work. Such topics are taught in order to equip neighborhood volunteers with the capacity to intervene early in local disputes, to create a safe place for expression and resolution of such conflicts, to reduce the potential of violence, and to enhance the quality of daily life at the neighborhood level.

This model spread rapidly within the criminal justice system. By the 1990s, Rogers, Kanrich, and Steinhouser (1990) reported that 1,500 citizen volunteers were active in community dispute resolution throughout New York State alone. They were donating their time, energy, and experience to conciliating, mediating, and arbitrating thousands of criminal and civil disputes a year!

As described above, this San Francisco initiative also gave birth to a curriculum for teaching conflict resolution to fourth grade children in the public schools (Davis 1983).

### Peace Courses at the University Level

Over the last decade, a number of universities in North America, England, and Europe have begun to offer fully accredited academic courses in peacemaking and/or conflict resolution (I. Harris 1988; Wein 1984). One, George Mason University of Fairfax, Virginia, offers a master's degree and a doctorate in this field. I advocate that such courses be offered at all schools of social work in all countries.

The curriculum should include lessons in theory, information gathering or research, examples of conflict resolution interventions, supervised field practice, the reading of recommended texts, written assignments, feedback procedures that increase self-awareness, and examinations.

During the first years of any such conflict resolution program, seminars and courses might be offered in the following areas:

*Theory Courses*

1. *Introduction to conflict resolution.* After learning basic concepts and definitions from the behavioral sciences, students look into causes and types of conflict, stages of escalation, some strategies for resolving conflicts, and some ways to rehabilitate conflict victims (Burton 1991; Chetkow-Yanoov 1987 and 1991; Deutsch 1973; Eisler 1987; Purnell 1988).

This course serves as prerequisite for all other studies in this field.

2. *Theories of human violence and potential.* In order to explore whether human beings are inherently violent, the concepts "aggression" and "assertiveness" are reviewed in biological, theological, and anthropological sources. Definitions of human nature are examined according to the values embedded in religion, psychology, Shakespeare, and a contemporary philosopher.

3. *Victimization and persisting conflicts.* Theories of crisis and victimization suggest that rage and revenge are at the core of continuing conflicts. This course examines these ideas, and suggests a range of therapeutic interventions that could help individuals, small groups, and ethnic populations achieve release from victim behaviors. Such release is seen as a necessary prelude to being able to function effectively as parties in any conflict resolution negotiations.

4. *Philosophy and methods of conflict research.* Research literature is surveyed in order to apply relevant technologies to gathering data about conflict situations, monitoring interventions systematically, and evaluating the effectiveness of efforts made to resolve conflicts. Research sophistication is also required to test a number of hypotheses about conflict dynamics and escalation.

5. *Special colloquium.* This forum would be used to introduce students to experts in the field from other university departments or visitors from abroad. They could, for example, listen to the wisdom of persons who have been engaged in the Middle East peace talks, or to United Nations personnel who negotiated the cease fire in Namibia. Students also investigate modern applications of traditional conflict resolution practices such as the Jewish *Din Torah*, the Arab *Sulcha*, or the Hawaiian practice of *Ho'onoponopono*.

*Courses in Practice*

6. *Skills and techniques for resolving conflicts.* This course parallels the above introductory one in theory. Students first explore the principles of conflict de-escalation, basing their efforts in a number of conflict models. Selected principles of mediation, arbitration, negotiation, and treaty making are taught as applied skills, through games, simulations, and fieldwork experiences in a variety of life settings (Bickmore 1984; Lingas 1988; Weingarten and Leas 1987).

This course serves as a prerequisite for all other practice studies in the field.

7. *Alternative dispute resolution (ADR).* This seminar examines a number of dispute-resolution formats that can serve as alternatives for adversarial court trial (or civic litigation). Students take a beginning look at such alternative methods as negotiation, bargaining, arbitration, trial by peers, victim-offender mediations, etc. The seminar includes lectures, simulation exercises, videotaping, and presentations from expert practitioners of ADR.

8. *Small group processes in negotiation and mediation.* This seminar demonstrates the relevance of small group process to conflict resolution technologies—especially to basic processes of mediation (Chandler 1985; Northen 1969). The seminar includes some of the theory and skill essentials of negotiation in small groups, and exposes students to the implications of small-group negotiations in family, labor relations, international, global environmental, and other settings.

9. *Computer-assisted intercultural meetings.* Based on the work done in Israel, the class examines a curriculum of lessons that teaches coexistence facts, attitudes, and skills in pairs of computer-linked schools–and concludes with a hosting and visiting experience at the end of the school year. Students examine various applications of this format and are encouraged to develop similar computer-based pedagogic programs.

*Special Fields of Conflict Resolution*

10. *Women and men in a changing society.* As Israel, located among the traditional societies of the Middle East, changes into a modern posturban society, students examine the changing roles of women and men in the family, in the professions, in politics/government, and in society generally. Developments such as the feminist movement will be studied and evaluated.

11. *Religious-secular dialogue.* As Israel becomes a modern country, it will have to find ways to serve the needs of both its traditional orthodox and its modern secular citizens. This course will look for ways to lessen religious-secular (and parallel right/left) tensions. A number of suggested interventions, including encounter dialogue meetings, will be studied and evaluated. New ways will be explored for loving our neighbors as ourselves.

12. *Intergroup relations.* As citizens in a pluralistic Israeli society, students are introduced to the many ethnically different Jewish and Arab-Palestinian groups living in the country itself, and in the Middle East generally. A review of intergroup relations in Israel over the past decades follows. The course includes experiencing an encounter with representatives of another group, and discussions of how all parts of Israeli society might start to practice the basics of coexistence.

13. *Labor relations.* This course provides background knowledge about labor-management relations in Israel and abroad–both in the public and in the private sectors. It focuses on labor negotiating collective bargaining agreements, grievance procedures, minority rights, and managing the problems of

retrenchment or technological change. Lectures are supplemented with in-class role-plays and small-group mock sessions.
14. *Teaching conflict resolution in the public schools*. This course focuses on the utilization of social work knowledge in grade and high school curricula of peace studies. Basic principles of social change, unlearning and re-learning habits, human nature, and trust building will be tailored to the needs of teachers, pupils, and parents. Participants will also review a range of interventions for making the administration of specific schools sufficiently flexible and democratic so that conflict resolution can be taught in a supportive atmosphere.

After the first full year, and in accordance with an evaluation of results, courses should be adjusted to make them more effective. Also, presuming that the evaluation proves basically positive, the following three years can be devoted to developing such additional interdisciplinary offerings as:

* Theological traditions and peacemaking.
* Limits of the earth: Applying conflict resolution technologies to physical environment and human ecology issues.
* Democracy in a pluralistic or multicultural society.
* Images of peace in utopian communities, literature, and the performing arts.
* The role of communications media in conflict and peacemaking.
* Alternative futures and citizen action.
* Directed reading and research.

Certainly, enough options are possible in order to offer a major in conflict resolution (Lundy 1987; Walton 1969).

### Communicating Creatively in the Midst of Conflict

Human beings of all ages, when caught up in conflict situations, can learn a way of communicating that can help them de-escalate the conflict. This process can be used by families in conflict, in labor-management disputes, by motorists in a collision, children from rival schools, secular humanists who clash with deeply religious believers, leftists who scream at rightists, neighborhood citizens who fight with City Hall bureaucrats, street gangs, rival ethnic groups, or feuding neighbors–if they are ready to change old habits.

In many countries today, groups and individuals are learning a process evolved by Dr. Marshall Rosenberg, an American psychologist. He developed what he calls a "Giraffe" or compassionate way of responding to anger and violence. When threatened by an upset person, instead of reacting with anger, blaming, or counterviolence, we can learn to give silent respect to our own emotions and then try to understand the feelings and unmet needs of our opponent (i.e., empathize with whatever might be causing them to explode at us). This process breaks the vicious circle of escalating conflict, releasing energies to get our own needs met in a way that also meets the needs of our opponent. Giraffe is equally helpful when we want to initiate a nonviolent confrontation with someone else.

People who have learned Giraffe are able to respond compassionately to one another. Responding in this way requires a high level of self-awareness and a willingness to learn how to be empathic. Empathy means deliberately projecting our consciousness (by means of imagination and fantasy) into the situation and feelings of another person, in order to understand what pain or passion might be making them behave as they do. We can empathize without losing our own identity, without becoming overidentified with the other person, and without accepting the other person's behavior.

Since many upset people generate conflict because of their own vulnerability or frustration, receiving compassion and empathy often enables them to feel safe enough to deal with difficult issues nonviolently. Clearly, the offering of empathy is unconditional, is not judgmental, does not limit the other's range of choices, and does not include arguments about who has "the facts" right.

The basic framework for such (compassionate) communication involves four steps.

1. As a Giraffe person, we first *describe the behavior that we find disturbing* in objective rather than judgmental language ("My father says that I cannot buy a motorcycle . . .").
2. We then *express the feelings* that we experience in relation to what we have just observed ("I feel sad and disappointed . . .").
3. Next we *describe the needs and desires* out of which our feelings have emerged. In other words, our needs affect both

what we observe and our feelings relating to such events ("I would have liked to be independent regarding my transportation needs . . .").

4. Finally, we *request the specific action(s)* that would allow our desires to be fulfilled. If people sometimes contribute to our discomfort (or prevent our needs from being fulfilled), we can request a change in their behavior. These requests should express what we want, rather than what we do not want, and also be stated in non-judgmental terms ("I'd like him to tell me what I could do to show that I am responsible enough to own a motorcycle . . .").

To put the Giraffe process into effect, several preconditions are usually necessary. First, we need training, and opportunities to practice, the newly learned empathy skills in our daily lives. We need to feel secure, and that other important people in our lives support us. Workbooks and audiovisual aids are available for learning the basics, but these are best practiced in small group settings with an experienced leader. Such a guided group experience seems essential for playing Giraffe roles, as well as for giving and receiving feedback (Green 1990; Rosenberg 1983).

## *IMPLICATIONS*

The above curriculum models are based on social science principles relevant to motivation, human nature, social change, unlearning and relearning habits, and trust building. They are meant to enable learners to develop simultaneously at the intellectual, the emotional-attitudinal, and the action-skills levels. Also, the program is meant to be applicable to events and norms indigenous to the country in which they are taught.

Participants are expected to learn to be responsible for their own behavior, to define "strength" in both physical and nonphysical terms, and to apply these in their own lives (Bickmore 1984; Kreidler 1984). Similarly, teachers who have learned to speak in the Giraffe way might serve as role models for the pupils in their classrooms, in the school yard, and in the neighborhood around the school.

Actually, the teachings described in this chapter are based on an assumption—that it is possible to educate all age groups toward greater psychological and political maturity. In the UNESCO bulletin titled *Features* (Derksen 1982), such maturity is operationalized to mean that we become human beings who can:

1. Stop analyzing problematic situations in terms of who is right or wrong (i.e., innocent or guilty).
2. Learn to recognize the relativity of our own viewpoint.
3. Become aware of the difference between facts and opinions, as well as show sensitivity to the norms and opinions of others.
4. Analyze the causes of a conflict, and what might be making it escalate.
5. Recognize, and become capable of coping with, our own aggressiveness—especially when we are under tension or pressure.
6. Learn to handle personal conflicts in nonviolent ways (e.g., by listening and dialoguing, by expressing empathy, or by bargaining).
7. Act as an informal facilitator or mediator among our friends and peers.
8. Overcome the tendency to resist change, especially if it means I have to change some of my habits or my cherished beliefs.

We should be trying to produce human beings who are flexible, happy with their own identity, and capable of appreciating others for their unique qualities—in an increasingly pluralist world.

Peace learning can also be reinforced by a positive educational climate. Well-organized schools, increasingly open to democratic patterns of educating and ready to cooperate with other agencies, are essential for the success of education for peaceful living. Peacemaking knowledge, attitudes, and skills, like those of reading or mathematics, should be taught and retaught several times during a person's learning career. The continuum of conflict resolution might start in nursery, with the three chairs format as well as the songs and folkdances of other peoples. Learning to speak and read several languages follows. Fourth grade pupils should experience being "conflict managers." In junior and senior high schools, peacemaking courses can include formal academic content, and be supplemented with educationally focused encounter meetings with members of another group or culture. Courses taught at universities would strengthen the thrust with audiences of adults, and might be supplemented by continuing-education programs for retirees.

The above teachings should be reinforced by programs and articles in the mass media, in popular music, in the theatre, and in both fiction and nonfiction literature. In fact, the time has come for us to merchandise our accumulated experiences, insights, and generalizations about conflict resolution in "packages" that can be learned by normal people in all walks of life in all countries.

We must make sophisticated efforts to press beyond the status quo, to make plans to influence social policy, and to strive for the emergence of well-informed public opinion. The implementing of peace education cannot be left to others.

## *SUMMARY*

This chapter reviewed what education and social work might contribute to the field of conflict resolution. It assumes that peacemaking attitudes and skills can be identified and taught. They should be part of the curriculum of all public schools and universities in every country. The rest of the chapter described a diversity of available conflict resolution curricula geared for nursery school, grade school, junior high school, high school, university student, and adult learners.

# Chapter 10

# Summary and Recommendations

Earlier in this book, I claimed that certain levels of conflict are healthy, and may well spur the participants to take risks, become more creative, or make greater conciliatory efforts. These kinds of conflict stay within the norms of acceptable behavior, and the opponents remain open to the option that their conflict can eventually be resolved. As we are able to identify human and environmental factors that impede or enhance conflict resolution, third-party interventions will become more effective.

## *FACTORS THAT IMPEDE CONFLICT RESOLUTION*

Conflicts seem to get worse under certain conditions. Some of the factors that make conflicts escalate, or interfere with efforts to resolve existing conflicts, are summarized below:

1. In situations where rivals feel that a desirable outcome or prize (such as owning diamonds or winning an Oscar) is not available to everyone, competition is likely to intensify greatly;
2. When rivals are in each other's immediate proximity (such as the fans of two football teams in the same stadium, or fanatics from different political parties on the same street corner), their disagreement is likely to escalate into violence;
3. Whenever the amount of communication between opposed groups lessens (often because one side is convinced that there is no one to talk to on the other side), differences tend to harden and the conflict escalates;

4. When the number of participants in a conflict grows (e.g., from a small committee to a large crowd of protesters), the likelihood of losing control, as well as of escalation, increases;
5. When a community lacks normative rituals or third-party structures for dealing with local conflicts, small disagreements tend to escalate into large ones;
6. When differences between parties become focused on personal characteristics of the participants (especially if they feel their honor or existence threatened) rather than on the issues, the conflict tends to escalate.
7. Conflicts in which local leaders are challenged in the law courts or in the news media are likely to escalate from normative adversary procedures into norm-violation and violence; and
8. When a conflict has so dichotomized a community that bystanders must choose between one side or the other, the conflict is likely to escalate further.

According to principles advocated in this book, a conflict will probably escalate when:

9. Conditions of crisis or tension continue over a long period of time;
10. Parties in a conflict experience strong emotions (such as fear, jealousy, guilt, desire for revenge) and tend toward ideological or psychological closedness;
11. Power or resources available to the parties in the conflict are asymmetrical; and
12. Weak groups feel excluded from participation, and conclude that decision making regarding their welfare is arbitrary and coercive.

There is a high probability that people who grew up in environments full of suspicion, fear, anger, and/or violence will be pessimistic about human nature and cynical about anything ever changing. When they did try to solve local problems or to resolve conflicts between neighbors, they got burned. After years of frustration, their "learned powerlessness" gradually reduces them to such survival tactics as selfishness or apathy. Feeling isolated and helpless, they are likely to huddle within their own group rather than communicate with people or groups unlike themselves. Such social closedness seems useful for self-protection against victimizers who lurk in the environment. However, ethnic closedness is often at the root of conflicts that escalate into blaming, lashing back, abusing the human rights of minority groups, or trying to destroy those who become designated as the enemy.

## FACTORS THAT ENHANCE CONFLICT RESOLUTION

People who have grown up in a supportive environment, have experienced loving/empathic care, and were socialized into values and skills enabling them to cooperate with their neighbors, are not likely to get caught up in drawn-out conflicts or violent wars.* People who have also engaged in successful social action tend toward an optimistic definition of human nature and are likely to know many ways of countering the negative factors listed above. Their approach to conflict resolution would include:

1. a basic trust in process and in intergroup dialogue;
2. analysis (i.e., diagnosis) of the causes of behavior;
3. an ethical use of power—e.g., to strengthen the weaker party in an unbalanced power situation;
4. fostering mutual respect among conflict participants;
5. keeping lines of communication open between feuding groups;
6. utilizing buffer arrangements to keep rival hotheads apart (especially in the initial stages of a conflict);
7. working with small groups of delegates or leaders rather than with large crowds;
8. making special efforts to keep conflicts short;
9. using a range of strategies to open up a closed social system;
10. encouraging processes of participatory decision making;
11. preventing the personalization of a conflict;

---

*Although it is beyond the scope of this book, today's archeologists are writing about "partnership cultures" that lived in peace for thousands of years (Eisler 1987, Jeter 1989).

12. avoiding the use of adversary procedures; and
13. avoiding any dichotomization of the environment in which a conflict is raging.

Conflict escalation can also be prevented by clarifying whether traditional ways of managing conflicts still exist and utilizing them. Reconciliations or settlements based on win/win rather than win/lose outcomes should be promoted by experienced third-party professionals and well-trained volunteers.

## A SYSTEMS MODEL OF THE CONFLICT RESOLUTION FIELD

I see conflict revolution as overlapping with two other major areas of human endeavor: therapy and education (see Figure 10.1).

When conflict resolution borrows from therapy, it generates processes of individual and group healing that must precede mediation between bitter enemies (enabling, for example, apologies and forgiveness in situations of long-term victimization). Conflict resolution linked with education makes theory-derived knowledge and applied skills available to its practitioners. Finally, the linking of education and therapy enriches conflict resolution by equipping us to deal with value changes. When these three large disciplines work well together, we are equipped to bring about the systemic transformation so essential for conflict resolution to be effective.

Figure 10.2 suggests the actual complexity of its predecessor.

### The Helping Professions

In order to achieve prenegotiation outcomes such as healing or conciliation, we must take lessons from such helping professions as pastoral counseling, marriage counseling, social work, psychology, political psychology, or social psychiatry. As mentioned above, when victimizers can apologize and victims can forgive, conflict resolution can get underway.

### Educators

The teaching of theory-based knowledge and of practice skills involves the contribution of academics (professors and researchers)

FIGURE 10.1. Three Major Components of Conflict Transformation

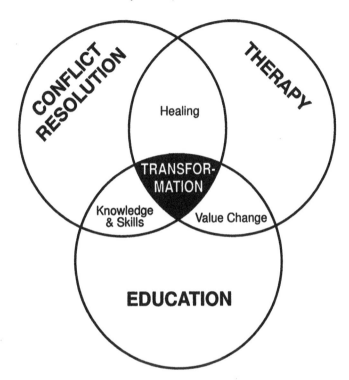

as well as practitioners (public and private schoolteachers). Reporters and communicators from the mass media have much to contribute to the distribution and popularization of knowledge. Some have also been known to implement mediation roles effectively, especially if employed by nongovernmental organizations (NGOs) such as universities or commercial television networks.

### Conflict Resolvers

Professionals in this field attempt to contain conflicts (i.e., to prevent them from escalating into violence), to make the conflict duration as short as possible, and to achieve transformation by means of a variety of conflict resolution technologies (such as buffering, facilitating, healing, mediating, advocacy, arbitration, and treaty administration). These efforts, though done in a multitrack

FIGURE 10.2. A Second Look at Components of Conflict Transformation

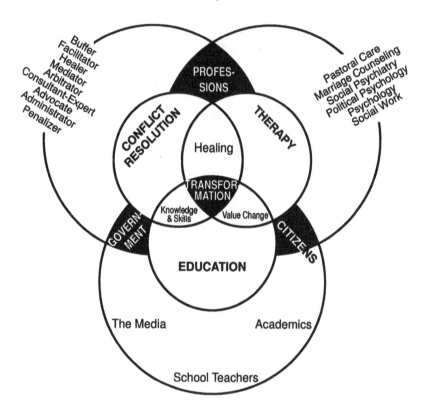

format, are usually compatible with the official work of (Track 1) governmental institutions and services.

## RECOMMENDATIONS

According to this model, enlightened citizens who wish to achieve de-escalation of a conflict should make such specific invest-ments as are listed here:

1. As is being done experimentally in some parts of Australia, Hawaii, Israel, Canada, and the United States, citizens should insist that: (a) all school-age children, starting at the kindergar-

ten level, be taught objective information about other ethnic groups living in their region and have opportunities to encounter each other in structured educational situations throughout the grade and high school years; (b) parallel programs should be set up for their parents—who will have to deal with their own ignorance, anger, and fear (Chetkow-Yanoov 1985; Wein 1984); (c) all curricula should include a cleansing of textbooks and films of bigoted stereotypes; (d) sensitive training programs, often funded by voluntary contributions, should be set up each year for classroom personnel who are to teach innovative curriculum content.

2. Similarly, we might express our concern by lobbying, in every country, for a national policy which ensures that all children be taught two or three languages. This policy, if implemented all over the world, would expose each child to other cultures and other value-based worldviews, as well as help them realize that their group, as unique as it is, is but one of many significant ones on earth.

3. In situations of asymmetric power or status, citizen movements can demand and monitor interventions appropriate to strengthening the weaker side, and to putting limits on the overly strong. Eventually, after resources have become more symmetric, the two sides can be helped to seek win/win resolutions for their conflict situation.

4. We should devote specific efforts to encourage participatory styles of decision making at home, in our schools, and in the workplace. In this connection, human beings from all walks of life must learn how to encourage open (or two-way) flows of communication and feedback. Increased communication between contending parties lessens the power of rumors and stereotypes, makes for increased trust, and is essential to the resolution of conflicts.

5. All citizens and voluntary groups should become skilled in keeping conflict situations as short as possible. The longer a conflict lasts, the more likely both sides are to suffer from some degree of burnout, victimization, or self-hatred. When capacities to cope are reduced in these ways, conflict is likely to escalate rapidly.

6. Human beings of all ages should have the opportunity to learn and to practice, in their everyday lives, some mediation or bargaining skills, simple ways for sharing resources (or cooperation), as well as techniques for listening to their own feelings as well as to those expressed by others (Brager and Jarin 1969; Chandler 1985; Edelson 1981; Fisher and Ury 1983). Pragmatic incentives should be innovated for rewarding citizens and colleagues who are willing to improve their conflict-management habits rather than continue obsolete practices such as complaining, blaming others, shouting, or resorting to violence.

7. Concerned citizens, as well as members of the helping professions, should join together in coalitions to lobby for reduction of governmental spending on armaments and military activities. In such social action, they could bear witness to the suffering due to continuing poverty, illiteracy, or unemployment–and insist that budgets be refocused toward social programs. Such efforts contribute not only to the rethinking of our national priorities but also to the reduction of factors which cause conflicts to escalate (Schaffner-Goldberg and Rosen 1992)

8. Increasingly, citizen groups are expressing dissatisfaction about how mass media reports stress sensationalism at the expense of accuracy–often contributing to the escalation of a conflict with simplistic analysis and exaggerations meant to catch the viewer's attention. People interested in conflict resolution should find ways to enlist the media as partners in this enterprise. The Conflict Resolution Network (CRN) of Sydney, Australia, for example, sponsors media peace awards every year (Cornelius 1993). Others suggest that communication professionals can function as "media mediators," bringing contenders together by satellite conferencing in ways that resemble shuttle diplomacy but are much faster (Botes 1993). The media, with the assistance of skilled actors and writers of fiction stories, should also be utilized to teach basic facilitation or mediation skills in popular formats.

## *CODA*

Having an innovative idea (such as teaching peace skills) is vital, but it is not enough. We must also use our professional resources to go beyond the status quo, make daring social plans, and utilize all available resources to influence public policy.

If we retain the humility to admit our limitations, and if we remember to work together with the many groups and professional disciplines sharing our concern today, we should be able to stand up and be counted among those who "seek peace and pursue it" (Psalms 34:15).

# Bibliography

Addams, J. (1983). *Peace and Bread in Time of War* (1922). Silver Spring, MD: NASW Classics Series.

Alfi, Y. (1986). *Theatre and Community: Ways to Implement a Community Theatre.* Jerusalem: The Jewish Agency, in Hebrew.

Alinsky, S. D. (1946). *Reveille for Radicals.* Chicago: University of Chicago Press.

Altemeier, W. A., O'Connor, S., Sherrod, K. M., and Tucker, D. (1986). Outcome of abuse during childhood among pregnant lower income women. *Child Abuse and Neglect,* 10: 319-330.

Amir, Y. and Sharan, S. (Eds.). Others ( 1984). *School Desegregation: Cross-cultural Perspectives.* Hillsdale, NJ: Lawrence Erbai Associates.

Anda, D. (1984). Bicultural socialization: Factors affecting the minority experience. *Social Work,* 29, March-April: 101-107.

Andrews, A. B. (1991). Social work expert testimony regarding mitigation in capital sentencing proceedings. *Social Work,* 36, September: 440-445.

Atherton, C. R. (1990). A pragmatic defense of the welfare state against the ideological challenge from the right. *Social Work,* 35, January: 41-45.

Avruch, K. and Black, P. W. (1990). Ideas of human nature in contemporary conflict resolution theory. *Negotiation Journal,* 6, July: 221-228.

___ (1991). The culture question and conflict resolution. *Peace and Change,* 16, January: 22-45.

Baden, N. (1991). The victimization debate: Implications for conflict resolution. Paper for course "Conflict 695." *ICAR,* George Mason University, October 7.

Benedict, R. (1970). Synergy. *Psychology Today,* 4, June: 53-55, 74-77.

Bernstein, S. (1965). Conflict and group work. *Explorations in Group Work.* Boston University School of Social Work, 54-80.

Bickmore, K. (1984). *Alternatives to Violence: A Manual for Teaching Peacemaking to Youth and Adults.* Cleveland: Friends Meeting.

Bloom, L. Z. (1990). Reunion and reinterpretation: Group biography (of former Japanese prison-camp inmates) in process. *Biography,* 13, Summer: 222-234.

Botes, J. (1993). Television and conflict. *Conflict Resolution Notes,* 11, September: 26-27.

Boulding, E. (1990). The dialectics of peace. *The Dialectics and Economics of Peace.* Center for Conflict Analysis and Resolution of George Mason University, Occasional Paper No. 3: 1-9.

Brager, G. A. (1968). Advocacy and political behavior. *Social Work.* 13, April: 5-15.

____ and Jarin, V. (1969). Bargaining: A method in community change. *Social Work,* 14, October: 73-83.

____ and Specht, H. (1969). A perspective on tactics. *Community Organizing.* New York: Columbia University Press, 261-283.

Browne, A. and Finkelhor, D. (1986). Impact of child sexual abuse: A review of the research. *Psychological* Bulletin: 99: 66-77.

Bunyan, J. (1909). Pilgrim's *Progress* (1678, 1684). New York: Collier.

Burton, J. W. (1991). Conflict resolution as a political system (1988). *The Psychodynamics of International Relations, Vol. II* (71-92). Eds. V.D. Volkan, D.A. Julius, and J.V. Montville. New York: Lexington Books.

____ and Sandole, D. J. D. (1986). Generic theory: The basis of conflict resolution. *Negotiation Journal,* 2, October: 333-344.

Chandler, S. M. (1985). Mediation: Conjoint problem solving. *Social Work,* 30, July-August: 346-349.

Charney, I. (1990). Children of victims and victimizers. *Contemporary Family Therapy,* 12, October: 407-426.

Cheatham, A. (1988). Peaceful playgrounds. *Fellowship,* September: 12-15.

Chetkow, B. (1963). Can social workers stand up and be counted for peace? *Peace and Disarmament Newsletter,* National Association of Social Workers, August-October: 15-20.

____ (1967). Some factors influencing the utilization and impact of priority recommendations in community planning. *Social Service Review,* 41, September: 271-282.

____ (1968). So go fight city hall. *Neighborhood Organization for Community Action* (194-203). Ed. J. B. Turner. New York: National Association of Social Workers.

Chetkow-Yanoov, B. (1976). Conflict as the dynamics of power in the local community. *Social Work Today,* 7 (8): 238-240.

____ (1984). Social work and social action: Implications for the agency. *Habitat International,* 8: 127-139.

____ (1985). *The Pursuit of Peace:—A Curriculum Manual for Junior and Senior High School Teachers.* Haifa: "Partnership."

____ (1986). Improving Arab-Jewish relations in Israel: The role of voluntary organizations. *Social Development Issues,* 10, Spring: 56-70.

____ (1987). *Dealing with Conflict and Extremism.* Jerusalem: Joint (JDC) Israel.

____ (1988). Teaching peace to adults: Dare we practice what we preach with leaders and officials? *Toward a Renaissance of Humanity* (245-265). Ed. T. R. Carson. Edmonton (Canada): World Council for Curriculum and Instruction.

____ (1990). Three patterns of establishment/minority-group relations: Implications for conflict resolution. *Social Development Issues,* 12, Spring: 62-73.

____ (1991a). Teaching conflict resolution at schools of social work: A proposal. *International Social Work,* 34, January: 57-68.

____ (1991b). The role of volunteers in conflict resolution. *Journal of Social Work and Policy in Israel,* 4: 61-76.

___ (1992). *Social Work Practice: A Systems Approach.* Binghamton, New York: The Haworth Press.

___ and Nadler, S. (1978). Community social workers and political leaders in municipal settings in Israel. *Journal of Social Service Research,* 1: 357-373.

Chin, R. and Benne, K. D. (1969). General strategies for effective changes in human services. *The Planning of Change* (32-59). (1961). Eds. W. G. Bennis, K. D. Benne, and R. Chin. New York: Holt, Rinehart and Winston, Second Edition.

*Choices: A Unit on Conflict and Nuclear War* (1983). Washington, DC: National Education Association of the United States.

Clark, M. E. (1990). Meaningful social bonding as a universal human need. *Conflict: Human Needs Theory* (34-59). Ed. J. Burton. London: Macmillan Press.

Cohen, R. (1990). *Culture and Conflict in Egyptian-Israeli Relations.* Indianapolis: Indiana University Press.

Cornelius, S. (1993). CR and media on public issues. *CRN News,* September 7.

Cornelius, H. and Faire, S. (1989). *Everyone Can Win: How to Resolve Conflict.* Australia: Simon & Schuster.

Coser, L. A. (1956). *The Functions of Social Conflict.* Glencoe, IL: Free Press.

Cox, E. O. and Parsons, R. I. (1992). Senior-to-Senior Mediation Service Project. *The Gerontologist,* 32(3): 420-422.

Crane, J. (1986). Potential contributions of social work education to peace studies. *The (Canadian) Social Worker,* 54, Fall: 102-106.

Danieli, Y. (1985). The treatment and prevention of long-term effects and intergenerational transmission of victimization. *Trauma and its Wake: The Study and Treatment of Post-Traumatic Stress Disorders.* Ed. C. R. Figley. New York: Brunner/Mazel.

D'Antonio, W. V. (1966). Community leadership in an economic crisis. *American Journal of Sociology,* 71, May: 588-700.

Davies, J. C. (1969). The J-curve of rising and declining satisfactions as a cause of some great revolutions and a contained rebellion. *The History of Violence in Violence in America* (690-730). Eds. H. D. Graham and T. R. Gurr. New York: Bantam Books.

Davis, H. (1983). *The Conflict Managers Program: Teacher's Manual.* San Francisco: Community Boards, Center for Policy Training, July, Mimeographed.

Davis, L. V. and Hagen, J. L. (1992). The problem of wife abuse. *Social Work,* 37, January: 15-20.

Derksen, S. C. (1982). Education for survival. *Features: UNESCO Bulletin of the News Media,* 48, Mimeographed.

Dershowitz, B. (1994). *We Are All Winners: A Language Arts Guide to Getting Along with Others.* White Plains, NY: Competency Press.

Deutsch, M. (1973). *The Resolution of Conflict: Constructive and Destructive Processes.* New Haven, CT: Yale University Press.

Diamond, L. and McDonald, J. W. (1991). *Multi-Track Diplomacy.* Grinnell, IA: Iowa Peace Institute, Occasional Paper No. 3.

Dimsdale, J. E. (1980). *Survivors, Victims and Perpetrators.* New York: Hemisphere Publishers.

Draucker, C. B. (1992). *Counseling Survivors of Childhood Sexual Abuse.* London: Sage.

Durbach, E. (1993). South Africa and its neighbors. *Fellowship,* 59, April-May: 25-26.

Eaton, J. W. (1952). Controlled acculturation: A survival technique of the Hutterites. *American Sociological Review,* 17, June: 331-340.

Edelson, J. R. (1981). Teaching children to resolve conflict. *Social Work,* 26, November: 488-493.

Eisler, R. (1987). The essential difference: Crete, and memories of a lost age. *The Chalice and the Blade.* San Francisco: Harper & Row: 29-41, 133-155.

Epstein, I. (1970). Professional role orientation and (the use of) conflict strategies. *Social Work,* 15, October: 87-92.

Etzioni, A. (1975). An analytic classification. *A Comparative Analysis of Complex Organizations* (23-39). New York: Free Press.

Fattah, E.A. (1981). Becoming a victim: The victimization experience and its aftermath. *Victimology,* 6 (1): 29-47.

Figueira-McDonough, J. (1993). Policy practice: The neglected side of social work intervention. *Social Work,* 38(2): 179-188.

Fisher, R. and Brown, S. (1988). *Getting Together: Building a Relationship That Gets to YES.* Boston: Houghton Mifflin.

___ and Ury, W. (1983). *Getting to YES: Negotiating Agreement without Giving In.* New York: Penguin.

Fisk, S. T. and Taylor, S. E. (1984). *Social Cognition.* New York: Random House.

Frank, J. D. and Ascher, E. (1951). Corrective emotional experiences in group therapy. *American Journal of Psychiatry,* 108: 126-131.

Frazer, E.F. (1962). *Black Bourgeoise* (1957). New York: Collier Books.

Free, L. A. and Cantril, H. (1967). Self-identification as liberal or conservative. *The Political Beliefs of Americans* (41-50). New Brunswick, NJ: Rugters University Press.

Freudenstein, R. (1992). Communicative peace. *English Today,* 31, July: 3-8.

Fulghum, R. (1987). We learned it all in kindergarten (Condensed from the *Kansas City Times). Reader's Digest,* November: 147.

Germain, C. B. (1991). *Human Behavior in the Social Environment.* New York: Columbia University Press.

Getzel, G. S. (1988). *Violence: Prevention and Treatment in Groups.* Binghamton, NY: The Haworth Press.

Ghandi, Mahatma (1948). *Nonviolence in Peace and War.* Ahmedabad, India: Navajivan Publishing House.

Gidron, B. (1983). Sources of job satisfaction among service volunteers. *Journal of Voluntary Action Research,* 12, January-March: 20-35.

Goldberg, G. S. and Rosen, S. (1992). Disengaging the peace dividend. *Social Work,* 37, January: 87-93.

Goodbread, J. (1993). Process work and mainstream conflict resolution paradigms. *Journal of Process Oriented Psychology,* 5, Spring-Summer: 18-25.

Green, N. S. (1990). *The Giraffe Classroom.* Cleveland Heights, OH: Center for Nonviolent Communication.

Grier, W. H. and Cobbs, P. M. (1968). *Black Rage.* New York: Basic Books.

Halevi, Y. K. (1992). The bitter legacy of withdrawal (from Yamit). *The Jerusalem Reporter,* April 16: 8-12.

Hamilton, D. L. (Ed.). (1981). *Cognitive Processes in Stereotyping and Intergroup Behavior.* Hillsdale, NJ: Lawrence Erlbaum.

Hamilton, R. (1958). Put the "social" back in social work. *Canadian Welfare,* December 15: 208-213.

Hareven, A. (1983). Victimization: Some comments by an Israeli. *Political Psychology,* 4, March: 145-154.

Harkabi, Y. (1972). Hostility and the concept of the enemy. *Arab Attitudes to Israel* (113-170). Jerusalem: Israel Universities Press.

Harris, I. M. (1988). *Peace Education.* London: McFarland.

Harris, T. G. (1970). About Ruth Benedict and her lost manuscript. *Psychology Today,* 4, June: 51-52.

Herman, J. L., Russel, D., and Trocki, K. (1986). Long-term effects of incestuous abuse in childhood. *American Journal of Psychiatry,* 143: 1293-1296.

Hoffer, E. (1951). *The True Believer.* New York: Harper & Row.

Hoffman, J. E. (1982). Social identity and the readiness for social relations between Jews and Arabs in Israel. *Human Relations,* 35: 727-741.

Hudson, W. W. (1978). The debate (on measurement and treatment) continues. *Social Work,* 23, November: 518-519.

Humphrey, N. (1981). Four minutes to midnight (BBC Television Lecture). *The Listener,* October 29.

Jabour, H. D. (1993). Seeing the light, breaking bread with my enemy. *Jade News,* 23, January: 11-12.

Jeter, K. (1989). Partnership cultures. *Cross-cultural Perspectives on Families, Work, and Change* (275-289). Binghamton, NY: The Haworth Press.

Kalmakoff, S., Hargraves, S., Cynamon, H., and Witheford, J. (1986). *Conflict and Change–A Peace Education Curriculum.* New Westminster, Canada: Public Education for Peace Society (PEPS).

___ and Shaw, J. (1987). *Peer Conflict Resolution Through Creative Negotiation: A Curriculum for Grades 4 to 6.* New Westminster, Canada: Public Education for Peace Society (PEPS).

Katan, J. (1974). Community work and political parties during election campaigns. *Community Development Journal,* 9, April: 125-131.

Kaufman, J. and Zeigler, E. (1987). Do abused children become abusive parents? *American Journal of Orthopsychiatry,* 57(2): 186-192.

Kavic, L. J. and Nixon, G. B. (1978). *The 1200 Days: A Shattered Dream.* Coquitlam, B.C., Canada: Kaen Publishers.

Kelman, H. (1991). Interactive problem solving: The uses and limits of a therapeutic model for the resolution of international conflicts. *Psychodynamics of*

*International Relationships, Vol. II* (145-160). Eds. V. D. Volkan, D.A. Julius, and J. V. Montville. New York: Lexington Books.

____ and Hamilton, L. (1989). *Crimes of Obedience.* New Haven, CT: Yale University Press.

King, M. L. (1958). *Stride Toward Freedom.* New York: Harper.

Klein, D. C. (1992). Managing humiliation. *Journal of Primary Prevention,* 12: 255-268.

Kluckhohn, F. R. (1951). Dominant and variant cultural value orientations. *Social Welfare Forum* (97-113). New York: Columbia University Press.

Konopka, G. (1953). The application of social work principles to international relations. *Social Welfare Forum* (279-288). New York: Columbia University Press.

Knudsen-Hoffman, G. (1993). Victims and victimizers—mutual sorrow, mutual suffering. *Fellowship,* 59, March: 25-27.

Kosmin, B. (1979). Exclusion and opportunity. *Ethnicity at Work* (37-68). Ed. S. Wallman. London: Macmillan.

Kramer, R. M. (1969). Types of community conflict resolution. *Participation of the Poor* (167-187). Englewood Cliffs: Prentice-Hall.

Kramer, R. M. (1981). *Voluntary Agencies in the Welfare State.* Berkeley: University of California Press.

Kramer, R. M. (1985). The future of the voluntary agency in a mixed economy. *Journal of Applied Behavioral Science,* 21: 377-391.

Kreidler, W. J. (1984). *Creative Conflict Resolution: More Than 200 Activities for Keeping Peace in the Classroom.* Glenview, IL: Scott Foresman.

Lee, D. (1959). Are basic needs ultimate? *Freedom and Culture* (70-77). New York: Spectrum Books (Prentice Hall).

Levin, S. (1992). The role of forgiving in conflict resolution. Speech for International Week, George Mason University, April 8.

Levy, C. S. (1973). The value base of social work. *Journal of Education for Social Work,* 9, Winter: 34-42.

Lewin, K. (1948). Self-hatred among Jews. *Resolving Social* Conflicts (186-200). New York: Harper.

Lindblom, C. E. (1959). The science of "muddling through." *Public Administration Review,* 19, Spring: 79-88.

Lingas, L. G. (1988). Conflict resolution within family and community networks. *Nordic Journal of Social Work,* 8: 48-58.

Lundy, C. (1987). The role of social work in the peace movement. *The (Canadian) Social Worker,* 55, Summer: 61-65.

Maslow, A. H. (1954). *Motivation and Personality.* New York: Harper and Row.

____ (1968). *Towards a Psychology of Being* (Second Edition) (1962). New York: Van Nostrand.

McDonald, J. W. and Bendahmane, D.B. (Eds.). (1987). *Conflict Resolution: Track Two Diplomacy.* Washington, DC: U. S. Department of State.

Merton, R. K. (1957). *Social Theory and Social Structure* (Revised Edition). Glencoe, IL: The Free Press.

Miedzinski, K. (1992). Conflict styles. *Effective Dispute-Resolution Skills, Workshop Training Manual*. Auckland Park,South Africa: Independent Mediation Service of South Africa (IMSSA).

Miller, A. G. (1986). *The Obedience Experiments*. New York: Praeger.

Mindell, A. (1988). *The Dreambody in Relationships*. New York and London: Penguin-Akarna.

___ (1989). *Working with Global Problems*. New York and London: Penguin-Akarna.

Mitchell, C. (1990). Necessitous man and conflict resolution, *Conflict: Human Needs Theory* (149-176). Ed. J. Burton. London: Macmillan.

Montville, J. V. (1987). The arrow and the olive branch. *Conflict Resolution: Track Two Diplomacy* (5-20). Eds. J. W. McDonald and D. B. Bendahmane. Washington, DC: U. S. Department of State.

___ (1989a). *Conflict and Peacemaking in Multi-Ethnic Societies*. New York: Lexington Books.

___ (1989b). Psychoanalytic enlightenment and the greening of diplomacy. *Journal of the American Psychoanalytic Association*, 37(2): 177-192.

___ (1993). The healing function in political conflict resolution. *Conflict Resolution Theory and Practice* (112-127). Eds. D. J. Sandole and H. van der Merwe. Manchester, England: Manchester University Press.

___ and Davidson, W. D. (1981-1982). Foreign policy according to Freud. *Foreign Policy*, 45, Winter: 145-157.

Moreno, J. L. (1944). *Sociodrama: A Method for the Analysis of Social Conflicts*. New York: Beacon House.

Moyer, K. E. (1971). *The Physiology of Hostility*. Chicago: Markham.

Netting, F. E. and Hinds, H. N. (1984). Volunteer advocates in long-term care. *The Gerontologist*, 24 (1): 13-15.

Northen, H. (1969). *Social Work with Groups*. New York: Columbia University Press.

Parry. D. (1987). From intensity to intimacy. *One Earth*, 7, April-May: 16-18.

Parsloe, P. (1987). Getting to the heart of the matter. *Community Care*, August 13: 18-19.

Parsons, R. J. (1991). The mediator role in social work practice. *Social Work*, 36: 483-487.

Parsons, R. J., Hernandez, S. E., and Jorgensen, J. D. (1988). Integrated practice: A framework for problem solving. *Social Work*, 33, September-October: 417-421.

Pearson, J. and Thoennes, N. (1985). Mediation versus the courts in child custody cases. *Negotiation Journal*, 1, July: 235-244.

Peck, C. (1993). Rural southern voice for peace (RSVP): The Listening Project. *Fellowship*, 59, July-August: 17-19.

Pietila, H. (1982). New way of life–for whom and why? Unpublished paper at Seminar on The Quality of Life and Adult Education. Helsinki, October 20.

Purnell, D. (1988). Creative Conflict. *WCCI Forum*, 2, June: 30-52.

Pye, L. W. (1966). The roots of insurgency and the commencement of rebellion. *The Dynamics of Modern Society* (449-457). Ed. W. J. Goode. New York: Atherton Press.

Renner, C. E. (1994). Multicultural (peace-education) methodologies in second language acquisition. *Peace, Environment, and Education,* 3(17): 3-21.

Richan, W. C. (1991). Writing a brief about abortion. *Lobbying for Social Change* (108-717). Binghamton, NY: The Haworth Press.

Richmond, M. E. (1971). The case for the volunteer. *The Long View* (343-345) (1930). New York: Russell Sage, Brown Reprints.

Rittel, H. W. J. and Webber, M. M. (1973). Dilemmas in a general theory of planning. *Policy Sciences,* 4, June: 155-169.

Roderick, T. (1987-88). Johnny can learn to negotiate. *Educational Leadership,* 45, December-January: 87-90.

Rogers, C. R. (1965). Dealing with Psychological Tensions. *Journal of Applied Behavioural Science,* 1, January-March: 6-24.

___ and Ryback, G. (1984). One alternative to nuclear planetary suicide. *The Counseling Psychologist,* 12, September: 3-12.

Rogers, S. J. , Kanrich, S., and Steinhouser, I. (1990). *Understanding our Criminal Justice Volunteers: A Study of Community Mediators in New York State.* New York: Brooklyn Mediation Center.

Rosenberg, M. B. (1983). *A Model for Nonviolent Communication.* Philadelphia: New Society Publishers.

Rosenheck, R. (1985). Malignant post-Vietnam stress syndrome. *American Journal of Orthopsychiatry,* 55, April: 166-176.

Rosenheim, M. K. (1976). Notes on helping. *Social Service Review,* 50, June: 177-193.

Ross, M. G. and Lappin, B. W. (1967). The role of the professional worker. *Community Organization* (203-231) (1955). New York: Harper & Row.

Rothman, J. (1965). The Lewin formulation. *Minority Group Identification and Intergroup Relations.* Ann Arbor, MI: American Jewish Committee, 54-81.

___ (1974). Practitioner roles. *Planning and Organizing for Social Change* (35-60). New York: Columbia University Press.

Rothman, Jay (1989). Supplementing tradition: A theoretical and practical typology for international conflict management. *Negotiation Journal,* 5, July: 265-277.

Samooha, S. (1978). *Israel: Pluralism and Conflict.* London: Routledge and Kegan Paul.

Sanzenbach, P. (1989). Religion and social work. *Social Casework,* 70(9): 571-575.

Schaffner-Goldberg, G. and Rosen, S. (1992). Disengulfing the peace dividend. *Social Work,* 37, January: 87-93.

Schneiderman, L. (1965). A social action model for the social work practitioner. *Social Casework,* 46, October: 490-493.

Schottland, C. I. (1966). Administrative decisions and fund allocations in social welfare. *Economic Progress and Social Welfare* (65-91). Ed. L. H. Goodman. New York: Columbia University Press.

Seligman, M.E.P. (1975). *Helplessness.* San Francisco: W. H. Freeman.

Shamir, M. and Sullivan, J. L. (1985). Jews and Arabs in Israel: Everybody hates somebody, sometime. *Journal of Conflict Resolution,* 29, June: 283-305.

Shipler, D. K. (1986). *Arab and Jew: Wounded Spirits in a Promised Land.* New York: New York Times Books.

Shonholz, R. (1984). Neighborhood justice system. *Mediation Quarterly,* 5, September: 3-30.

Shook, E. V. (1985). *Ho'oponopono: . . . A Hawaiian Problem-Solving Process.* Honolulu: University of Hawaii Press.

Silverman, S. M. (1975). The victimizer: Recognition and character. *American Journal of Psychotherapy,* 39, January: 14-25.

Smoker, P., Davis, R., and Muske, B. (Eds.). (1990). Appendix: The Seville Statement on Violence. *Reader in Peace Studies* (221-223). New York: Pergamon Press.

Specht, H. (1969). Disruptive tactics. *Social Work,* 14, April: 5-15.

Stauffer E. R. (1987). *Unconditional Love and Forgiveness.* Burbank, CA: Triangle Publishers.

Steele, W. W. (1972). Understanding the adversary process. *Social Work,* 17, July: 108-109.

Susser, L. (1992). Controversial (Shulamit) Aloni is not out of the woods. *The Jerusalem Report,* October 22: 7.

____ (1993). History in the making: Peace breakthrough special report. *The Jerusalem Report.* September 23: 5-7.

Swartz, J. (1987). Palestinian editor urges negotiated peace. *The Ottawa Citizen,* December 2: A9.

Towle, C. (1965). *Common Human Needs.* New York: American Association of Social Workers.

Turnbull, M. (1975). Bennett pledges to free pensions from politics. *The Province Newspaper,* Vancouver, B.C., Canada, November 13: 13.

Viano, E.C. (Ed.). (1990). *The Victimology Handbook.* New York: Garland.

Volkan, V. D. (1988). *The Need to Have Enemies and Allies.* Northvale, NJ: Jason Aronson.

Wahlstrom, R. (1989). *Enemy Images and Peace Education.* Malmo, Sweden: School of Education, September, Miniprint No. 660.

Wallis, J. (1993). The "gang" summit: A report. *Conflict Resolution Notes,* 11, June: 11-13.

Walton, R. E. (1969). *Interpersonal Peace Making: Confrontations and Third Party Consultations.* Reading, MA: Addison-Wesley.

Warren, R. L. (1964). The Conflict Intersystem and the Change Agent. *Journal of Conflict Resolution,* 8, September: 231-241.

____ (1965). Types of purposive social change at the community level. Waltham, MA: Brandeis University Papers in Social Welfare, No. 11.

___ (1972). *The Community in America* (1963). Chicago: Rand McNally.

___ (1987). American Friends Service Committee mediation efforts in Germany and Korea. *Conflict Resolution: Track Two Diplomacy* (27-34). Eds. J. W. McDonald and D. B. Bendahmane. Washington, DC: U. S. Department of State.

___ and Hyman, H. H. (1966). Purposive community change in consensus and dissensus situations. *Community Mental Health Journal,* Winter: 293-300.

Watts, L. G. and Hughes, H. (1964). Portrait of a self-integrator. *Journal of Social Issues,* April: 103, 115.

Wein, B. J., Ed. (1984). World order education: Teacher training. *Peace and World Order Studies: A Curriculum Guide* (161-199). New York: World Policy Institute.

Weingarten, H. and Douvan, E. (1985). Male and female visions of mediation. *Negotiation Journal,* 1, October: 349-358.

___ and Leas, S. (1987). Levels of marital conflict: A guide to assessment and intervention in troubled marriages. *American Journal of Orthopsychiatry,* 57, July: 407-417.

Young, W. M. (1967). The case for urban integration. *Social Work,* 12, July: 12-17.

Younghusband, E. L. (1963). The challenge of social change. *International Social Work,* 6, April: 1-4.

Zak, M. (1992). *Walking the Tightrope: Encounters Between Jewish and Palestinian Youth in Israel.* Neve Shalom/Wahat Al-Salam: School for Peace.

# Index

Page numbers followed by the letter "t" indicate tables; those followed by "i" indicate illustrations.